The Data Worker's Injury Prevention Guide

By Deanna Aliano

Deanna Aliano, DeannaDYoga@gmail.com

The Data Worker's Injury Prevention Guide

Title ID: 9070801

ISBN-13: **978-1726275323**

Table of Contents

Dear Reader;

Desk jobs offer many unique challenges to our health and well-being. Our bodies were not meant to sit for extended periods of time, specifically not eight hours a day, five days a week. We were meant to move freely and openly, walking, climbing, stepping on varied surfaces and squatting. Technology has all but ensured we get less and less time outdoors, and more and more time with our rears in a chair.

Sitting all day takes its toll on our hips, lower back, neck and shoulders. It also doesn't do anything good for our circulation and lymphatic systems, which require movement to pump the fluids about our body, and to help eliminate the build-up of waste, contamination, and fat.

Staring at a computer screen is also shown to have negative effects on our eyes, shoulders, and neck. We have all experienced that awful tension headache brought on by leaning forward to read a screen, creating neck tension and eye strain.

Let's not forget about our hands, wrists, and forearms. Anyone who spends a lot of time at a computer is bound to know the feeling of stiffness and soreness that causes many to eventually change careers.

My hope with this book, is to offer some common sense preventative solutions to these problems. I also hope to light the way towards a few ways to relieve some of the common symptoms of overuse and misuse you may encounter.

This book is divided into five sections: The introduction- a general explanation of job related stress and injuries; ergonomic advice, to help you set yourself up in the best possible way to eliminate many common problems; job specific strength training, to help you develop task related strength which should allow for longevity and ease of function; relaxation and pain management, to show you some ways to alleviate job related stress, soreness and muscle tightness; and finally some suggestions on other services and recommendations that may be of use on your journey.

I hope these pages will be of great value to you. It is my wish that you are able to use this information to create more ease in your life, and therefor share that ease with those you pass along the way.

Remember, none of this will work if you don't put it to use!

Onward with the journey…

@DeannaDYoga

<u>Introduction</u>

The biggest complaints I see from people who work at computers all day are neck, shoulder, forearm/hands, and eye strain. This will likely not surprise anyone. These maladies are so common, in fact, I venture to say nearly anyone who has had to use a computer at all has experienced some of them.

Let's take a look at the anatomy of these problems, shall we?

We'll start at the top. The head weighs ten to eleven pounds. That's not to say the brain weighs that much - on the contrary; the brain only weighs about three pounds. The head consists of the brain, the skull, the eyes, the mouth and all those teeth. Imagine if you were to take a pole and put a human head on top of it, (I know, very morbid, but follow along). You have this tall pole and put a ten pound round rock on top of it. If you tip that rock even slightly in any direction, what is going to happen? It's going to lean and need counter balance to stay up. Now imagine you attached some rubber bands to the opposite side of the tipping, in order to stabilize it. What is going to happen to those rubber bands? They are going to stretch until they are at full tension (let's say they are not going to break for the sake of this discussion). Those rubber bands are going to lengthen, and lengthen, and then lengthen some more, until they are absolutely as long as they can go and still hold up that rock. Those rubber bands? They are your neck muscles.

Now imagine those rubber bands are constantly stretched to their maximum with that weight pulling on them. At some point there will begin to be some wear on those rubber bands. In terms of why we generally feel the soreness up close to the skull? Well ,those muscles attach to the skull right in that area; so not only are they strained, but that point where the heaviest weight is pulling on them is less pliable and made of a strong, fibrous substance. The fibers of the muscle near that attachment have to work extra hard to keep your head from falling off, and they are stretched and held in a static contraction (also called an isometric contraction). Those prolonged stresses on those fibers create tension because those muscles get used to being contracted and "forget" how to relax.

It's also helpful to note that the muscles in the front of the neck, the antagonist muscles, aren't actually being overworked as a result. They don't need to work against gravity.

So teaching those muscles in the back of the neck how to relax is an important part of the process of regaining balance and relieving tension headaches.

Moving down the neck into the upper shoulders, they are being affected by the muscles in the neck. That chain reaction along the upper back is all happening to keep the head from tumbling to the floor.

Continuing out into the shoulder blades, the trapezius muscle, the large muscles between your shoulders and neck that seem to be the source of all tension) attach into the top of the neck at the skull and down into the tops of the shoulder blades...so it may now be obvious why they seem to be a stress point. All the muscles that support the shoulder blades now have to work harder to fight the load brought down upon them from that head moving forward to look at the computer screen (or phone/book/desk/paperwork...). Having tightness in the shoulder blades can further send a chain reaction down the shoulders into one or both arms, continuing to the hands.

Now, if we focus on the hands and typing, we start another series of events, traveling back up to the neck and that stubborn trapezius muscle.

In order to type or use the mouse, our hands have to hover above the keyboard. Our fingers have to raise and lower onto the keys, using muscles that cross the wrist and attach into the forearm, near the elbow. Side to side movement of the hands at the wrist is needed to reach the keys, and some rotation and stabilization of the forearm is also necessary, which utilizes muscles that sit across the bones of the forearm, as well as cross the elbow and attach onto the humerus (upper arm bone). All of these muscles of the forearm can be deeply aggravated by a lot of typing, and, as mentioned above, can affect the upper arm, which attaches to the shoulder and shoulder blade… you see where this is going. It's all connected. There's not one easy fix to solving or preventing pain. It all needs to be taken into consideration when designing a program to strengthen muscles and prevent injuries.

The eyes present a more complex problem. While, yes, everything is connected, eye strain doesn't directly affect the postural muscles, however the strain on the eyes can absolutely contribute to neck issues by requiring the eyes to be closer to the screen. Eye muscles CAN be worked and strengthened, however it is not necessarily going to improve vision. It may, however help the eyes to feel better.

One final problem common among desk workers is lower back stiffness. This is mainly due to sitting position (and sitting in general) as sitting less than upright often creates rounding of the lower back, which has a similar effect as the pulling on the back of the neck (creating isometric contractions to hold the body up). Interestingly, having the head forward can have a chain reaction all the way down to the lower back (and beyond). Sitting also tends to keep the hip flexors in a shortened state and not in use, which is also a contributor in lower back stiffness.

While this book focuses mainly on upper back, arm and neck issues, we will offer some advice on relaxing the lower back.

Ergonomic Considerations

First and foremost, if you are lucky enough to have an opportunity to have a desk that can transform from a seated to standing position, that's the best case scenario. Being able to switch positions throughout the day will help alleviate some of the common problems of a desk job. If you do have the ability to stand at your desk, make sure the monitor is high enough (this goes for sitting as well - eye level), and spend the money on one of those wobble boards or some variation. Standing on a board or surface that moves a little will keep your muscles active, allow you to develop a stronger core, help stimulate your feet and ankles (go barefoot if you can), and help you continuously change positions as you work.

As mentioned above, the monitor should be at eye level and positioned so as to have the least amount of glare. This will help prevent neck and eye strain. It should also be close enough to read comfortably. One consideration is to change the fonts so that they are larger and easier to read.

The keyboard should be in a position that when you sit upright with elbows at your sides and bend your elbows 90°, the keyboard lands just under your hands. Ideally, this will happen when your chair height is adjusted correctly (see chair positioning section.). Consider getting an ergonomically correct keyboard. This allows for less wrist strain, and they are no more expensive than regular keyboards. Ergonomic keyboards can be used with a laptop, as well.

One interesting thing I don't see mentioned as much is the position and use of the mouse. If you are doing a lot of searches or copy and paste movement that you use a mouse for, it may be wise to find a way to reposition your mouse. There are some more ergonomic mice on the market, however the main problem is having to reach off to the side to use it, which puts a lot of strain on the rotators of the forearm...Mouse Strain. This soreness can be felt high in your forearm, near the elbow, and low down close to the wrist. If you are going to be utilizing the mouse a lot, perhaps position it closer to the keyboard, or even in front of it.

Chair position is pretty straight forward. Ideally, you should be situated so that when you are seated, your feet are flat on the floor, the knees are bent at 90°, as are your hips. If your feet don't touch the floor because of your height, the keyboard, or any other issue, it might be helpful to have a foot stool (or even some books or boxes) to put your feet on. They shouldn't be so high that your knees are higher than the seat, as that will translate into hip position and lower back pain. One gadget I have seen lately is a swinging foot stool that attaches to the underside of the desk, or a wobble board which allows foot movement as you sit. These may help to bring some movement into your body as you sit, so they may be a great idea! Just make sure when your feet are on them you are not compromising your ideal position. A good lumbar support is great to keep you from slouching.

Arm rests might seem like a good idea, however I find that most people use them to lean on which in turn pushes stress up into the shoulders and neck. I would use with caution and watch your habits.

Proper ergonomic set-up is imperative to keeping yourself pain free and creating longevity in

Ergonomic sitting for Data Entry.

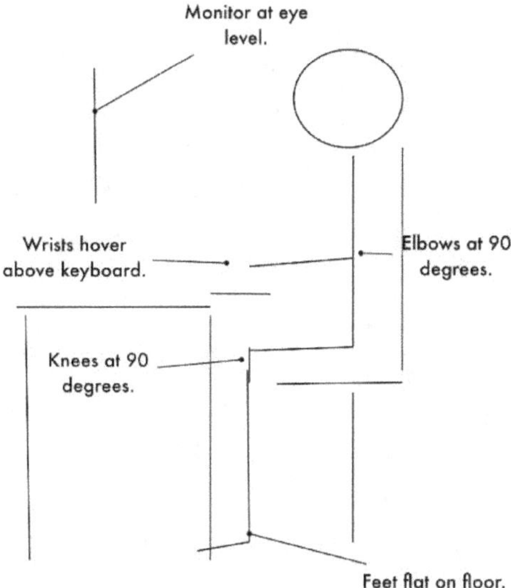

your job.

<u>Strength Training Exercises</u>

Using simple equipment, these exercises will give you an edge to preventing injuries. These exercises should be done several times a week, and should continue throughout your career. These are mostly smaller movements that can be done at your desk, or at home.

Equipment consists of exercise bands (begin with a thinner one and work up in thickness or double up as you get more proficient at the exercises), rubber bands (make sure they are not old so they don't break), a massage ball (or lacrosse ball), a Neckersizer cloth, a 4-5 inch massage ball, a roller, and small weights or a weighted ball (1lb to start). Also shown here is a taped up piece of yoga mat which can be used for finger exercises.

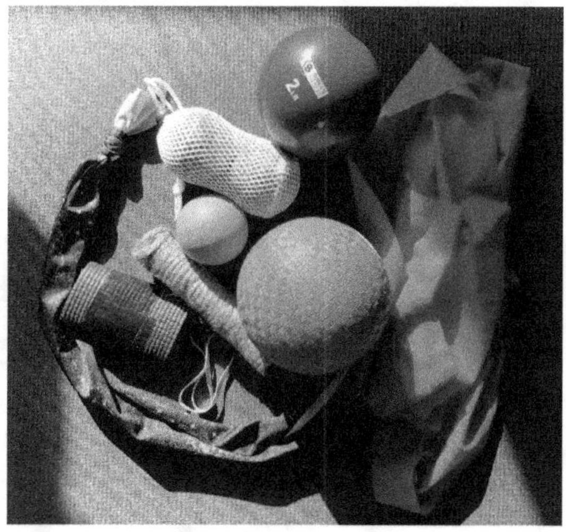

These exercises do not need to all be performed at the same time. Focus on one or two at a time, and spread them throughout the day as part of your wellness break (explained more in the last section of the book).

How many should you do? I prefer quality over quantity. Five reps performed well will offer far more benefit than fifteen reps performed badly. Being mindful in your movement practices will not only ensure that you are getting the optimal benefit for your physical body, but also give provide your mind with incredible benefits!

A gentle reminder that you should consult your physician before beginning any exercise program, and certainly if you have any injuries.

The Neck

Strength training the neck is vital to keeping many of the other injuries at bay. Remember that everything is connected, and the head weighs ten to eleven pounds. When the head isn't being held up properly, everything else gets affected.

Finding ways to engage the muscles in the back of the neck will help them to learn to work properly, and also relax. Remember, they tend to get stuck in static contractions a lot of the day, so show them some love with the following exercises, using the Neckercizer, or a soft, pliable cloth.

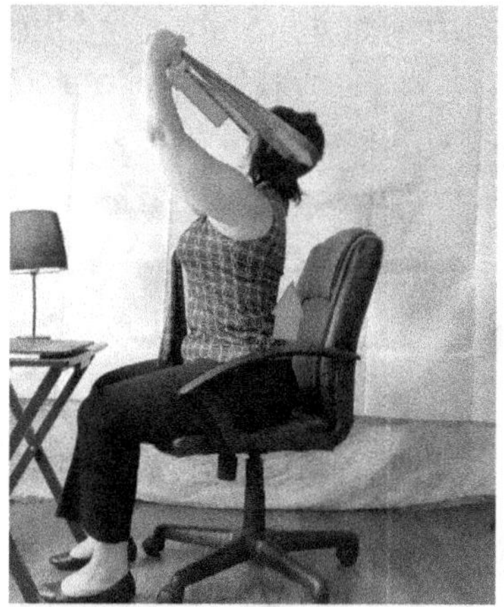

Begin by spreading out the fabric and placing it on the back of the skull. Sit tall, and grasp the knots. Begin to push your head back into the fabric as you resist with your hands.

This can also be done lying down, however I believe it is more effective seated and staying tall through the spine. Do five to eight repetitions.

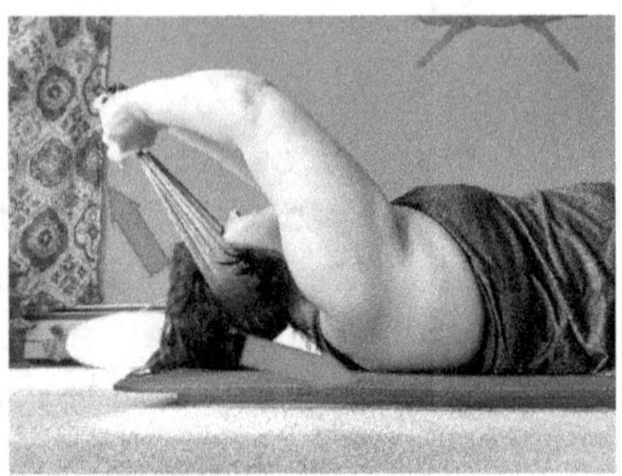

I recommend doing this exercise moderately until you know how it will feel for you.

In the same position with the fabric, now work to push the back of your head into the fabric while keeping your chin level to the floor. Repeat five to eight times, slowly with quality.

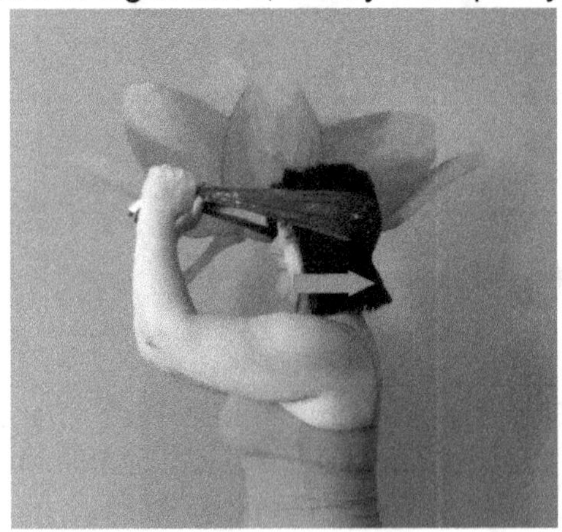

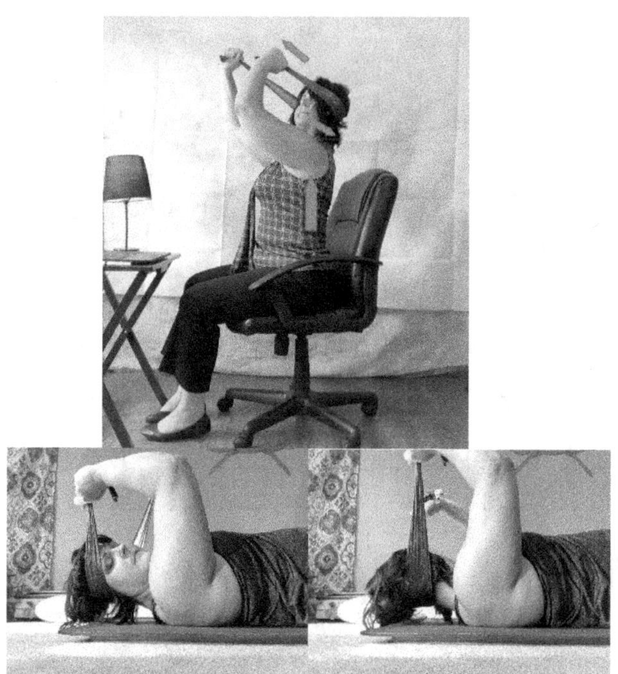

Next, holding the fabric in each hand, begin to twist the head side to side as you resist, pushing the back of your skull into the fabric. Use your hands to create as much or little tension as you want.

Repeat five to eight times each side.

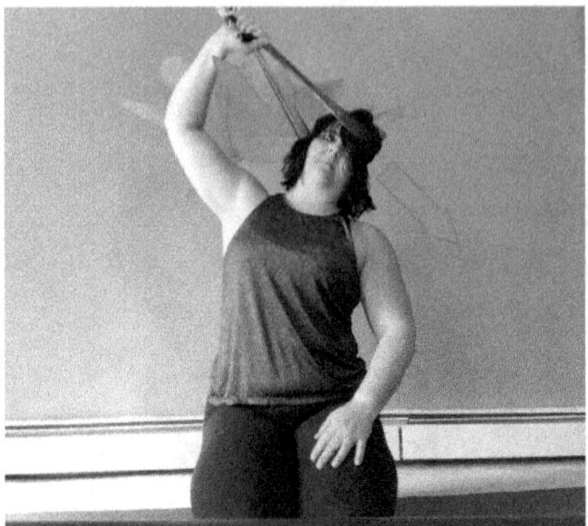

Now, holding the fabric in one hand off to the side, tilt your head into the fabric as you resist with your arm. Repeat five to eight times each side.

Shoulders

Strengthening the shoulder muscles, particularly the ones in the back, will assist your neck in holding the head upright. It will also assist in allowing the hands to move freely for typing.

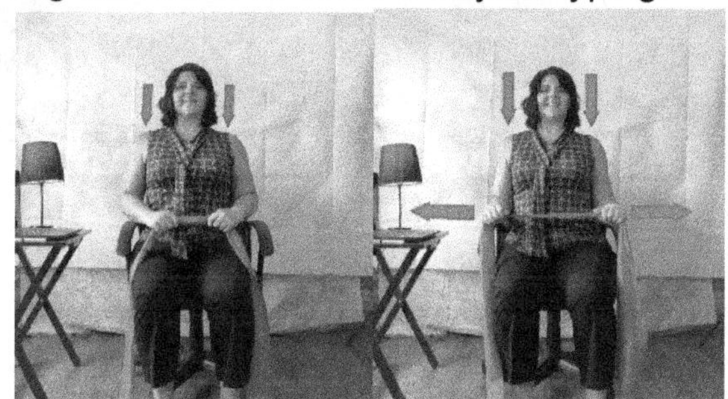

Using an exercise band, sit upright. Keep your shoulders down, away from the ears. Hold the band in front of your belly at elbow level. Keep your elbows at your side - they will not move during this exercise.

Pull the exercise band apart, as if you were going to rip it in two. Return and repeat.

This exercise can be done sitting on your knees, as well.

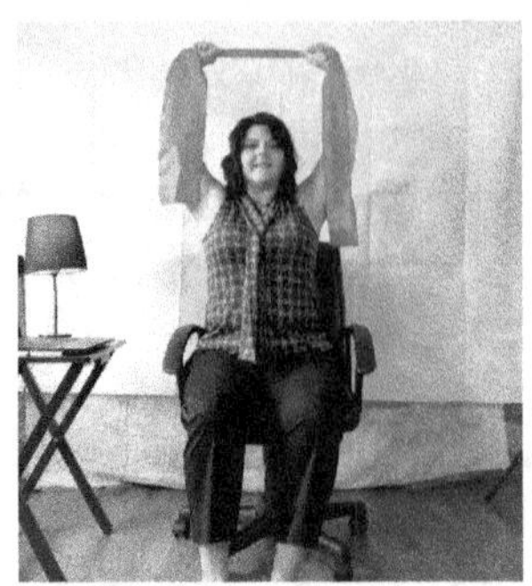 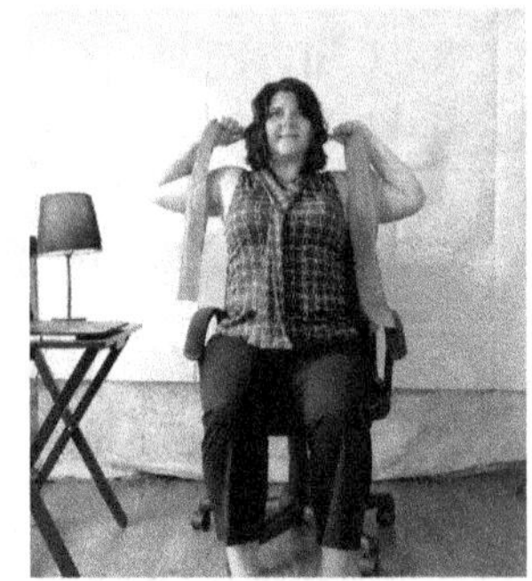

Hold the exercise band at a little less than shoulder width above your head. Pull it apart slightly as you pull it down behind your head, keeping the elbows bent and wide. Reach back up to start and repeat.

Below is a side view.

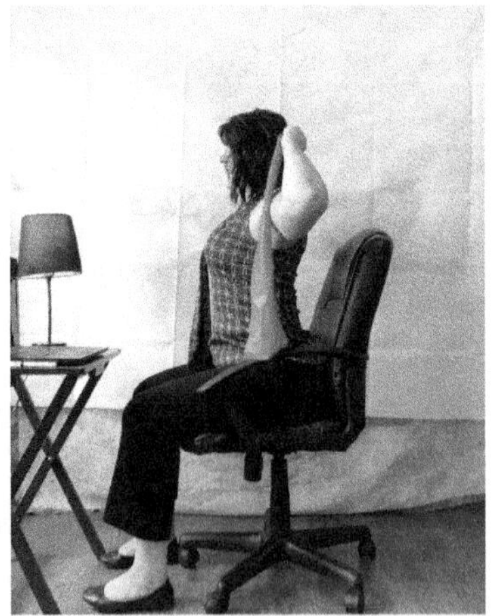

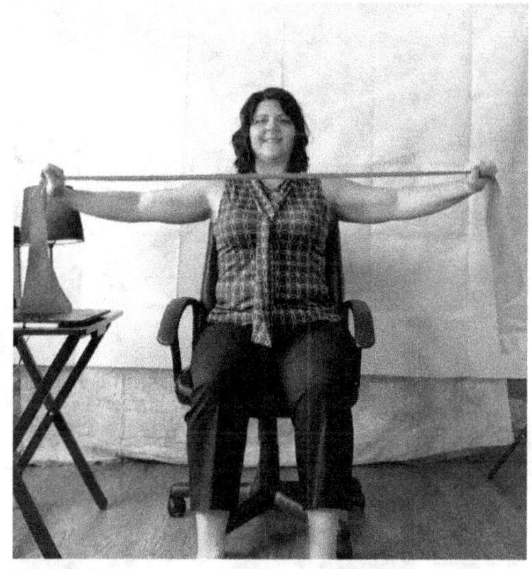

Hold the exercise band in front of your chest. Pull to stretch your arms out as far as they will go. Repeat.

You can also hold it out to tension and create small circles with the hands. This is a great deep strength builder, and also feels really good.

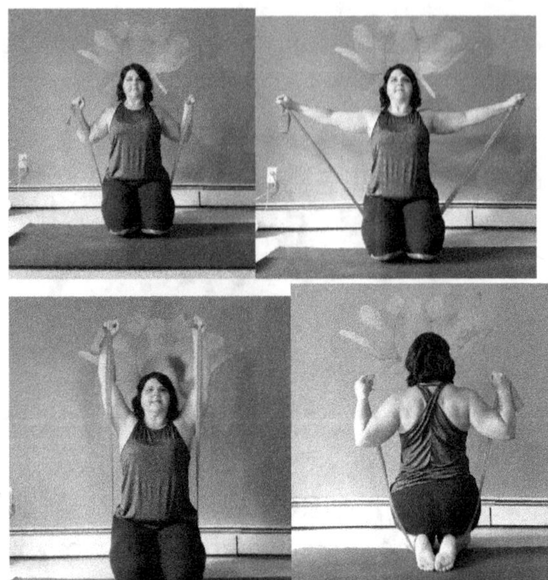

This next exercise is shown on the knees, however it can be done seated in a chair. Just sit on the center of the exercise band to keep it steady.

Sit on your knees and wrap the exercise band under your ankles. Start with elbows bent, hands up, holding the ends of the band. Press hands out long at your sides. Once there press up to the sky, then bend the elbows to come back to start. Repeat five to eight times.

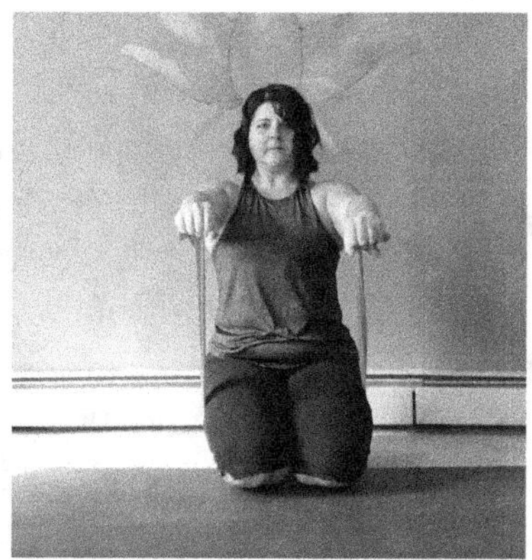

Some other things you can do from this position, are to pull the arms out in front of you into tension, and then all the way up to the sky (if you do not have any shoulder injuries).

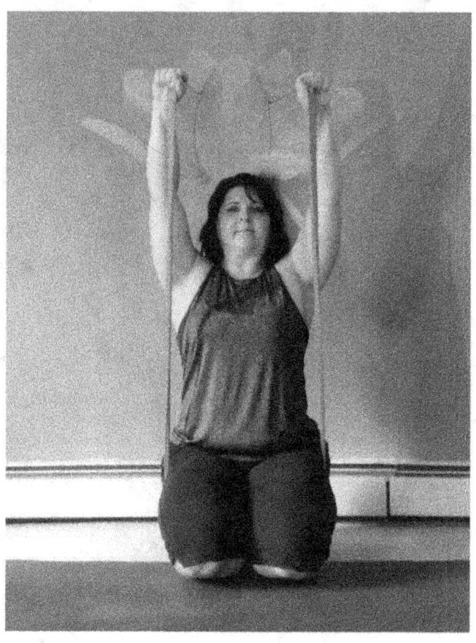

Forearm Strength

As mentioned in the introduction, forearms often are a unique problem for mouse users. These exercises will help you develop strength in the forearms, as well as down into the wrists and fingers. After all, the muscles of the fingers actually run up into the forearms!

You will notice I have used a small weight (in this case a weighted ball) for some exercise, and a band for others. Note that they can each be used for all of the exercises to build different types of strength. One caveat is the side to side movements of the wrists, which are better served with a band, in my opinion.

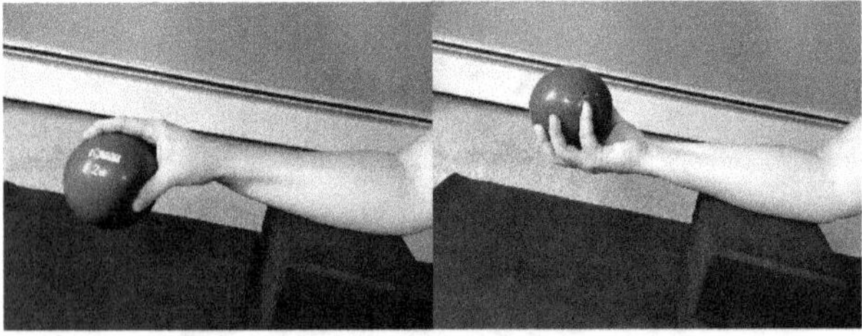

Hold the weighted ball or small weight in one hand. Rest the forearm on some yoga blocks or the side of a table. Turn the palm face down, then palm up. Rotate back and forth several times, taking your time.

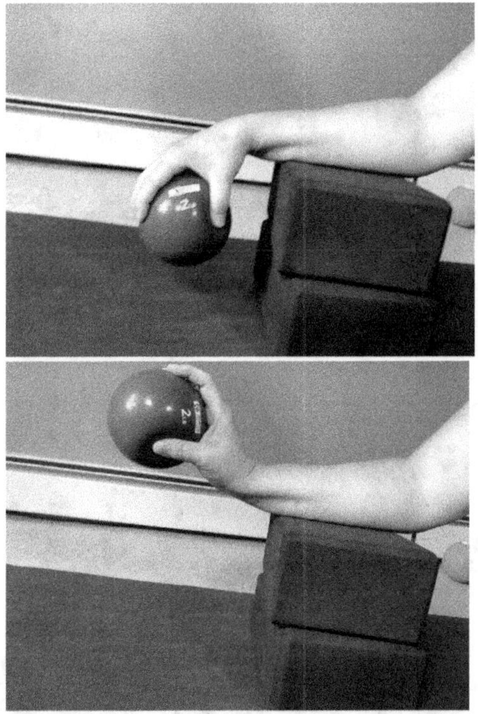

Now, holding the weight with the palm facing down, lift the weight as high as you can then back down.

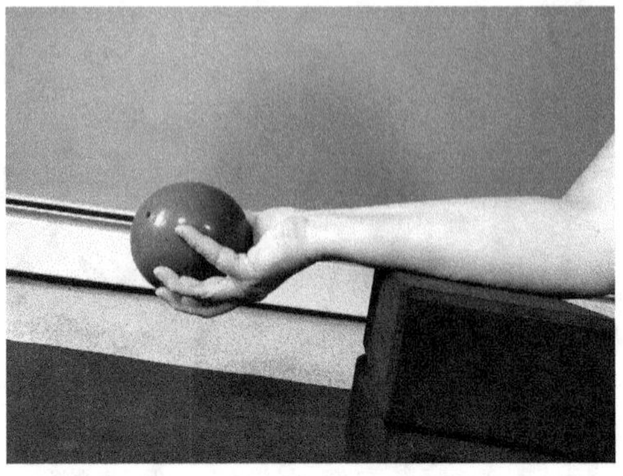

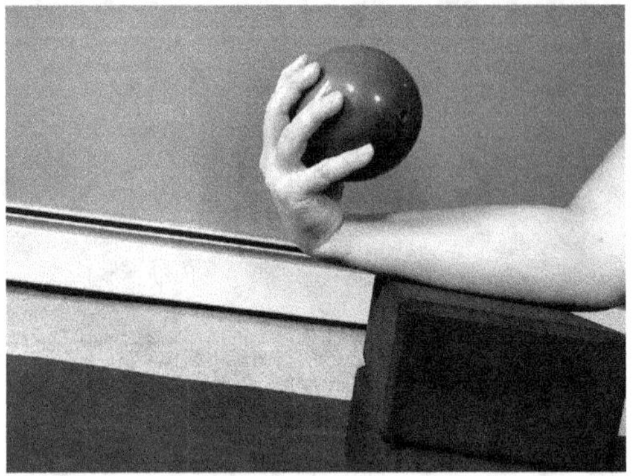

Now turn the palm face up and do the same. Note, this is not a bicep curl. All the work is in the wrist/forearm.

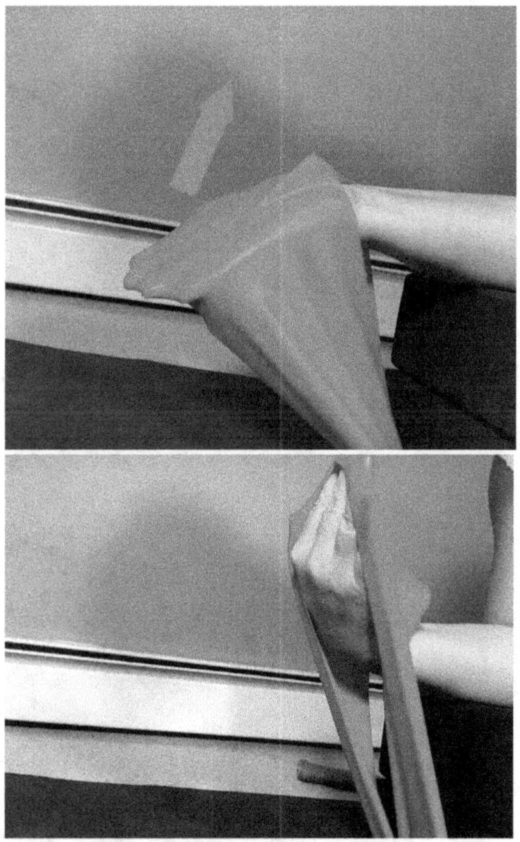

This is the same exercise with an exercise band. In these photos, I am kneeling on the ends of the band and extending and flexing into the wrists. Using the band allows the fingers to have more movement, thus creating a different type of resistance.

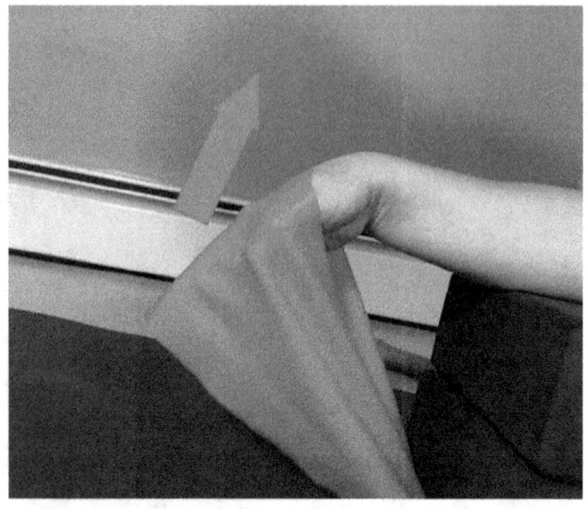

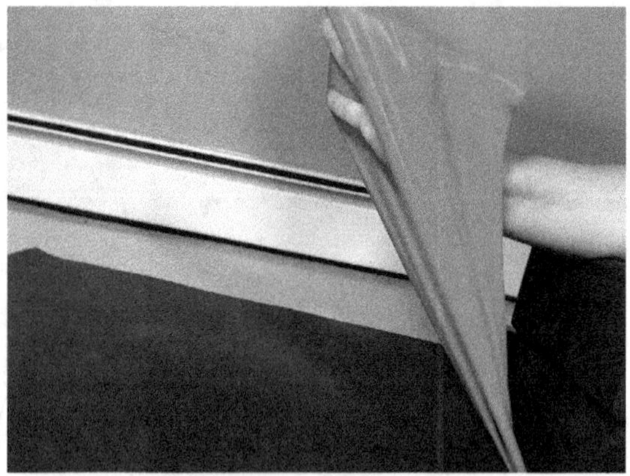

And this is the palm facing down variation.

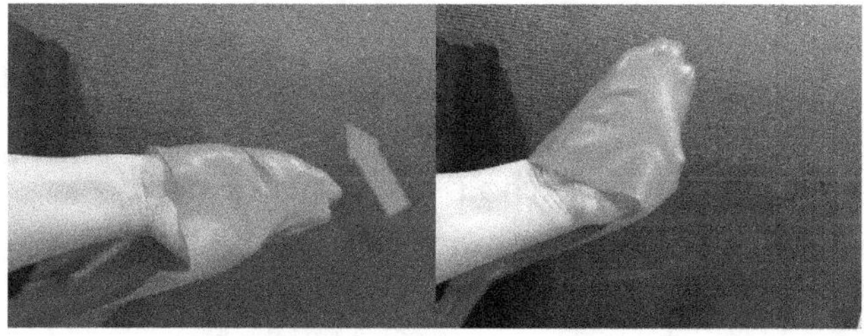

We can also work on lateral wrist movements by holding the band off to one side and pushing the hand into it. This is great work for typists.

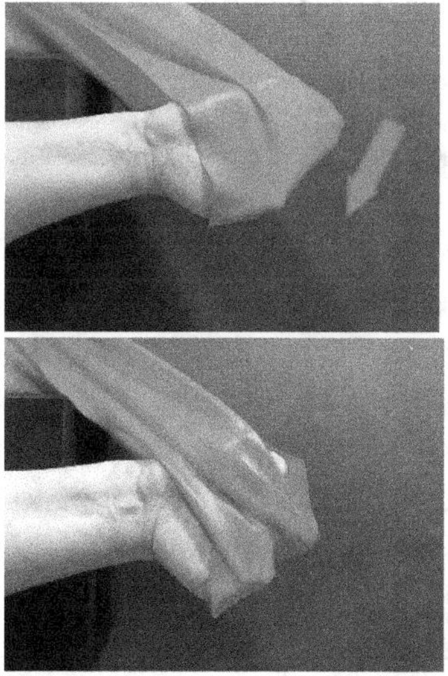

Fingers

We very rarely work our fingers, however it is essential for those who use them to create income. Keyboarding requires many levels of dexterity in the hands. Here are some exercises that can help strengthen the muscles that move the fingers.

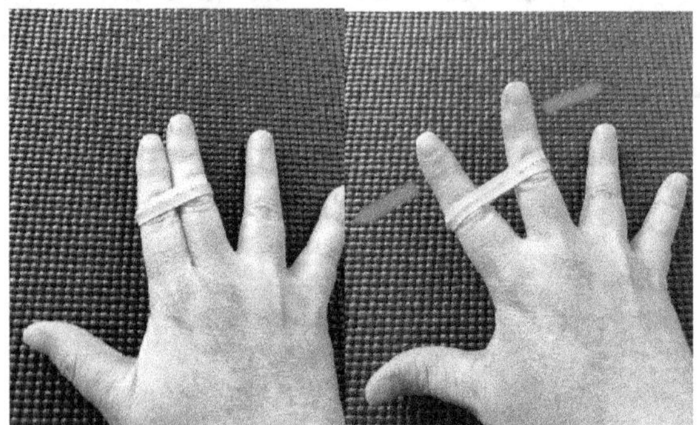

Most of these exercises use a simple tool that you probably have on your desk.

Place a rubber band around your pointer and middle finger at the mid-knuckle level. Make sure there is enough resistance by doubling it up until there is tension in the resting position. Then simply spread the fingers, release, and repeat.

Make sure you are using newer rubber bands that are not dried out and easily breakable. You can double up on the rubber bands for more resistance.

To continue, keep moving out to new fingers, as shown over the next page.

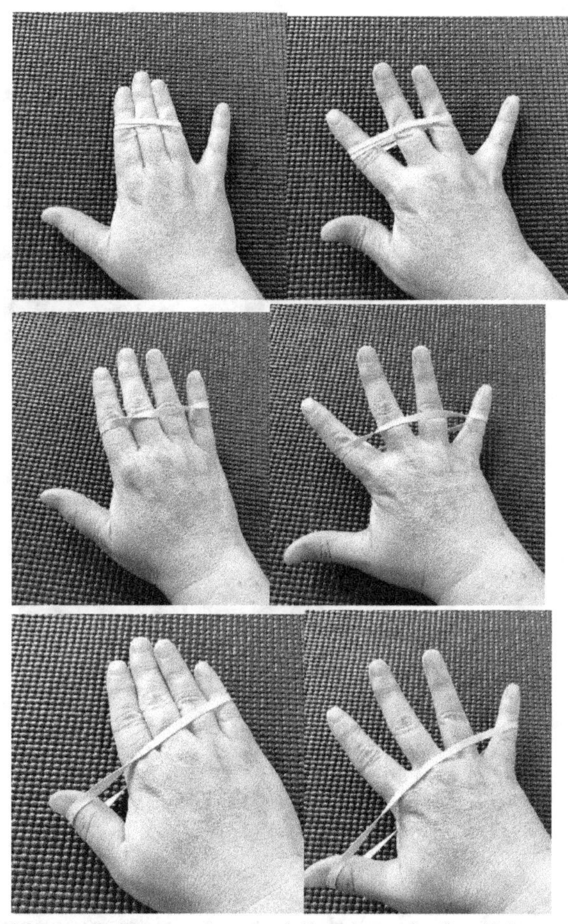

You might use two rubber bands for this one.

These next few exercises demonstrate some other rubber band strengtheners. These are performed by putting the rubber band on the pad of the finger, pulling back the opposite end and then pushing into the rubber band. Work each finger separately. These exercises are particularly useful for data entry workers.

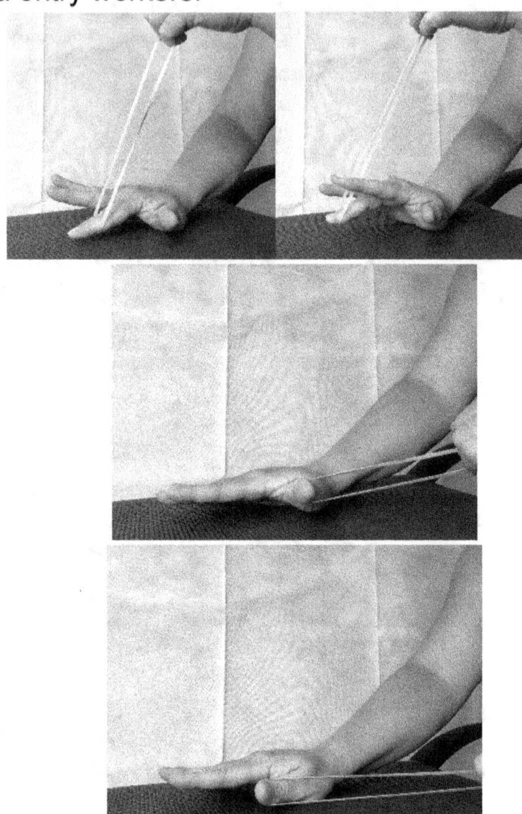

Now, work the opposite side- extension is important, too!

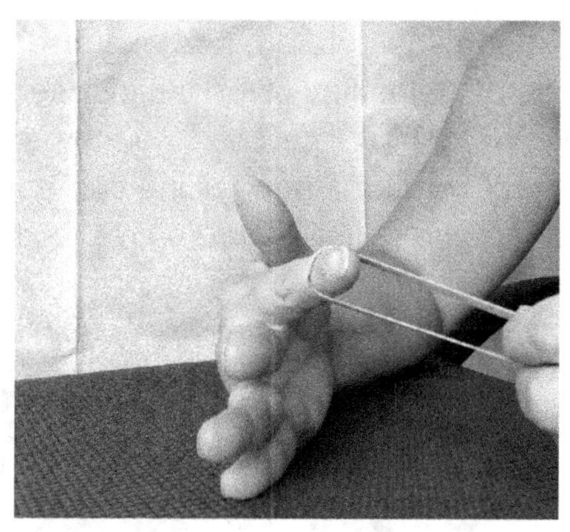

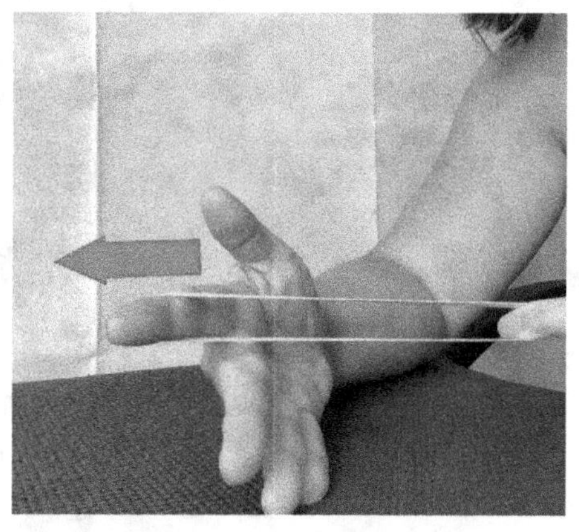

32

One final rubber band exercise that is particularly helpful involves putting the rubber band on the pad of the finger, placing the hand on a table in "tented" position, then pulling the resistance away from the finger as you "scratch" the finger towards your palm.

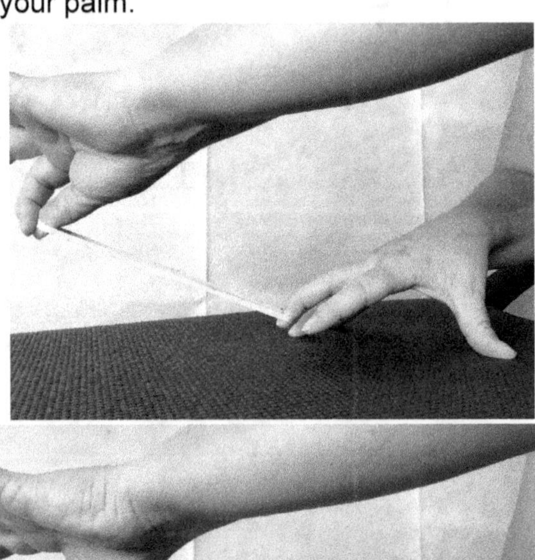

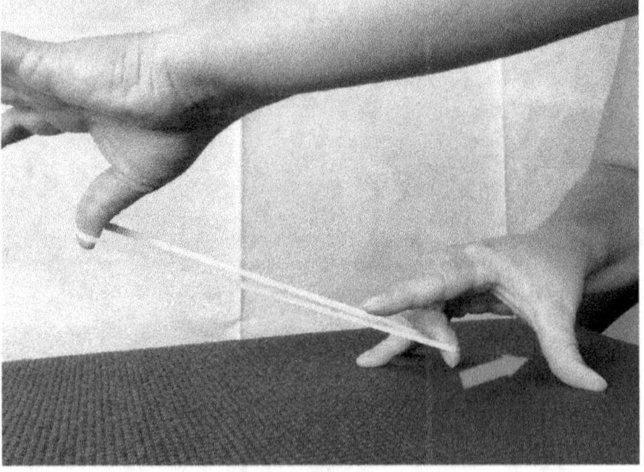

Repeat eight to ten times- QUALITY.

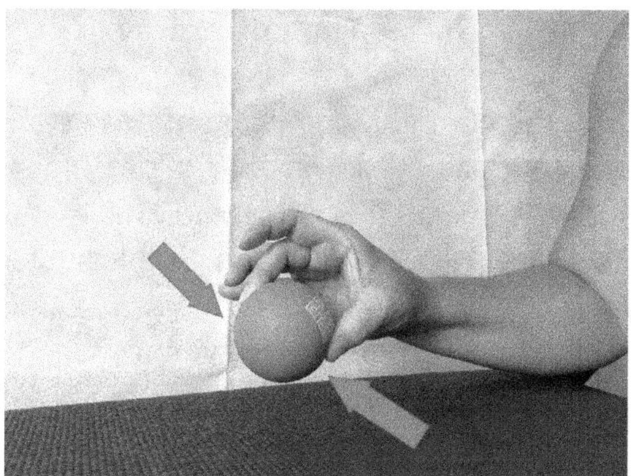

Another helpful exercise for the fingers/hands- take a small ball (here we have a lacrosse ball but it is a bit harder than need be) and place it between your thumb and each individual finger, squeezing and holding for a breath. You can use varying size balls a well as different hardness. You can also use a piece of rolled up yoga mat or other squishy material.

As you get stronger, finding other props will be useful.

The Lower Back

One common complaint of desk workers is lower back pain. While we will not get into extensive detail on this subject for this manual, I'd like to share a little information on this subject, as well as some simple solutions.

Desk jobs generally have us sitting all day. As many studies have recently pointed out, sitting is almost as bad for your health as cigarette smoking, and should be treated as a problem that should be rectified. Aside from the circulation issues that sitting creates, a large portion of lower back complaints can be traced back to extensive seated positions.

Several problems begin in our lower back when we are in a seated position all day. One very common problem is a chronic "rounding" of the lumbar spine. Similar to the problems in our neck muscles, the muscles in the lower back become exhausted from a constant static contraction. Over time, these muscles begin to disconnect from their job of stabilizing the lower back, and eventually develop a sort of temporary paralysis, no longer using that connection to the brain. This problem is far more common than we would think, and is actually quite easy to correct, although it does require constant work and a willingness to become aware of the problem.

One simple awareness exercise is as follows.

Pelvic Tilts with Activation (see next page for instructions).

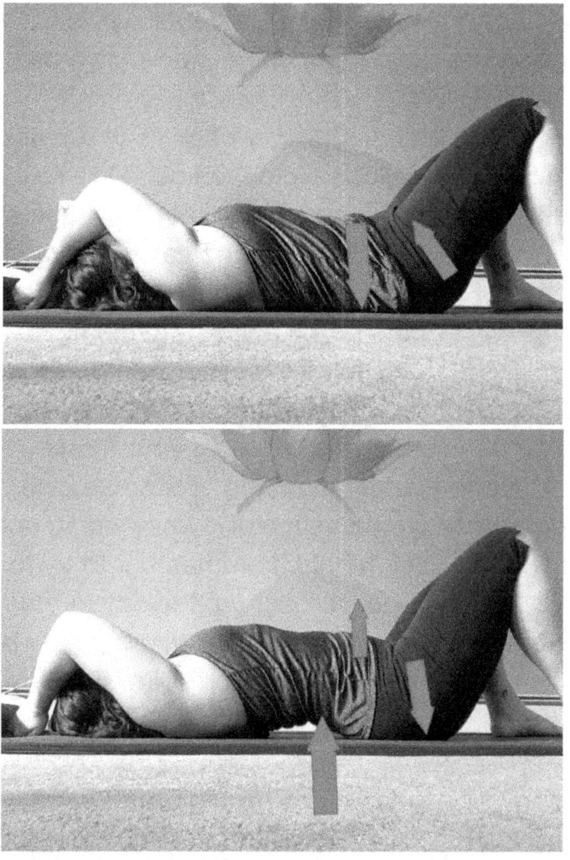

Lying on your back with your knees bent (or put your feet on a ball or in a sling), become aware of your lower back. Take one hand and slide the fingers under the lower back to see how much space you have between your back and the floor (if this isn't possible due to shoulder tightness it isn't essential).

Now, using your abdominal muscles (not your feet) pull your lower back into the floor (rounding). This action is a posterior pelvic tilt. You are tilting the top portion of the pelvis towards the floor.

Next, arch your lower back as you press the very tip of your tailbone into the floor. Do this with as much action as is needed to feel the muscles in your lower back- up into your rib cage- activate. This action is an anterior pelvic tilt. You are arching the top, front of the pelvis away from the floor.

Repeat this exercise several times as you begin to regulate your breath to the movement - inhaling as you arch, exhaling as your round.

Once you get the hang of this exercise, you will be able to do the action of it while sitting and standing. It will be helpful to remember to try to arch that lower back throughout the day to reset the position from sitting. This is also where it may be helpful to have a lumbar support pillow.

Hip Flexors

Another cause for lower back pain is our hip flexors. Our hip flexors, which attach into our lower back (lumbar spine), are continuously left in a passive, shortened position when we sit. Those muscles require strengthening and activation in order to stay healthy and pliable.

This exercise is one you can do with your office chair. If you are strong and used to this type of work, you may be able to do it without holding your desk, however, I recommend using the desk the first time, until you get the hang of it.

Stand facing your desk. Put your leg on the seat of the chair. If you are more flexible in the hips you can put your foot up on the back of the chair (with the knee on the seat), however it is not necessary unless you want a deeper quad stretch.

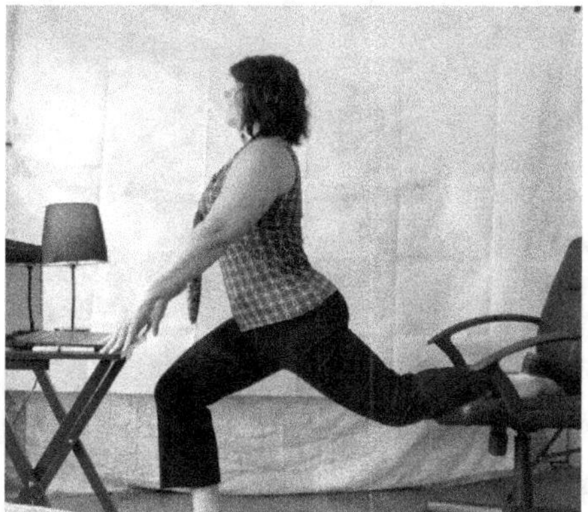

Keeping the ground foot still, and the knee over the ankle, slide the chair back into a lunge. Work to keep your hips square to the desk. This should feel like a nice stretch and you can come in and out of this a few times if you like.

Now, pull the chair/knee forward as if you are going to stand up. Instead of bringing the knee all the way forward, work to squeeze that hip forward into a slight posterior tilt (see last exercise). The goal here is to engage the hip flexors and get them active while stretching. You should feel like you are squeezing your glute on that side, as well as a little abdominal engagement (sort of a mini crunch).

Feel free to go in and out of this and the deeper stretch a few times. It will be nice to feel the stretch and activation a few times throughout your work day.

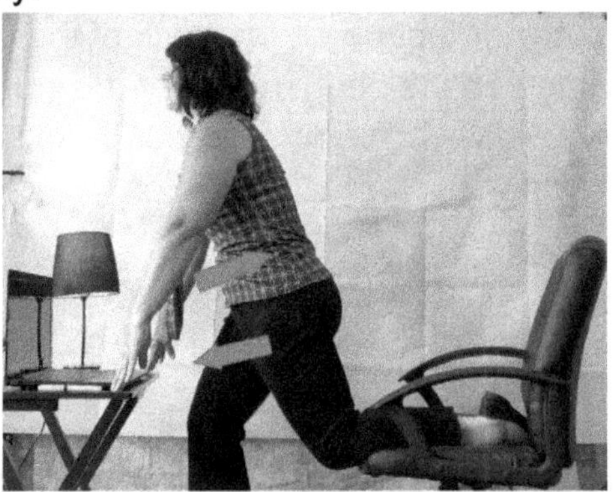

The above exercise can be done on the floor with your knee on a towel (if you have a hardwood floor) or some furniture movers (if you have a carpet). Work to keep the chest up, and possibly find a desk or chair to help steady your movements.

Eyes

Yes, eyes. Our eyes take a lot of abuse in these days of computers, smartphones, television… There are constant challenges to our eyes and they are something we don't often take care of.

Wearing proper eyewear can certainly help, but we can do more to keep our eyes healthy and help to prevent eye strain.

The next pages offer a few exercises you can do to strengthen the muscles of your eyes. They may not change your vision, but they can't hurt to work on!

Working on focusing the eyes at differing distances is a helpful practice. If we spend much of our day looking at a computer screen that is always the same distance in front of us, our eyes don't get the opportunity to change focus.

Sit up tall and bring your thumb close to your nose. Focus your eyes on your thumbnail.

Slowly move your thumb farther and farther away as you maintain focus, then bring it back in.

Repeat this a couple of times.

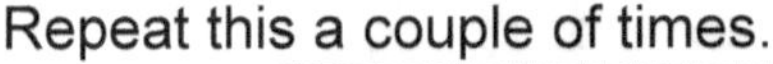

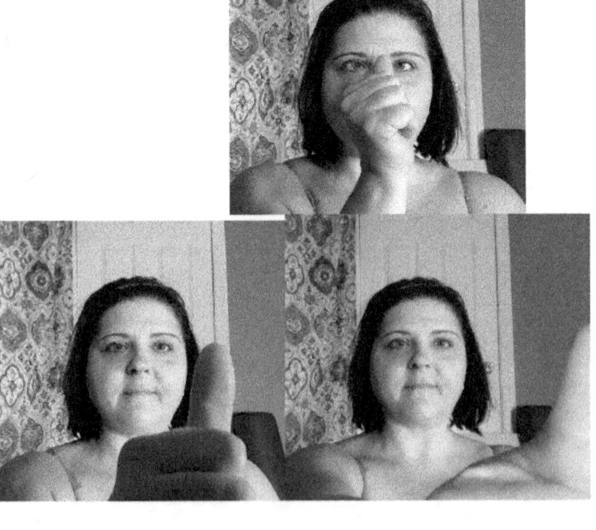

Eyes are meant to work in many directions. The muscles that move the eyes need exercise, just like all the others in the body. When we sit in one place and stare at a screen all day, they don't have to work as hard.

Sit up tall and gently, slowly take the eyes on a complete trip around their perimeter. Make sure to go both directions a couple of times a day.

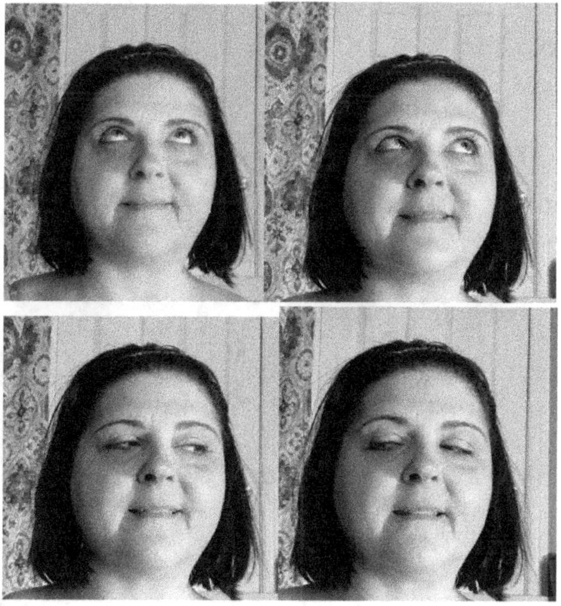

One final eye exercise is for peripheral vision.

Sit up tall and take a colorful object off to one side of your face. Look straight forward, and see how far back you can go before losing sight of the object. Work to see if you can increase that awareness over time.

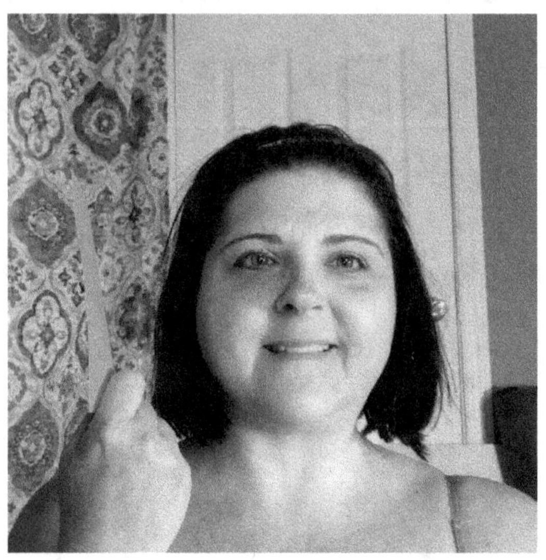

<u>Relaxation and Management</u>

Exercising and strength training problem areas are essential to keeping injuries at bay and giving you career longevity, however, what should you do if you do become stiff or sore?

First, make sure there isn't an existing injury. The only way to ensure this is to see your doctor and make sure there are no issues that would precede these relaxation exercises. If you are only experiencing minor, occasional stiffness, chances are there are no serious injuries and the following activities will be wonderful. If your pain is more than occasional, you should make sure there are no disc issues or ligament damage before proceeding. If your doctor does suggest there is more extensive injuries, show him these exercises to determine if they would be of benefit or you.

The first few stretches/movements are things you can do at work (or home) using your desk chair.

Torso/Twists

A simple twist is always a great way to feel good in the middle of the day. It should be noted that this may not be recommended for those with disc issues, so please remember to check with your doctor.

Begin by sitting up tall facing the front. Take your arm to the back of your chair (if that is an option for you - if not just bring it around to the side) and begin to twist to that side. Take the opposite hand to the arm rest if there is one and use it for gentle leverage.

Remember to maintain a tall spine while twisting, and do both sides.

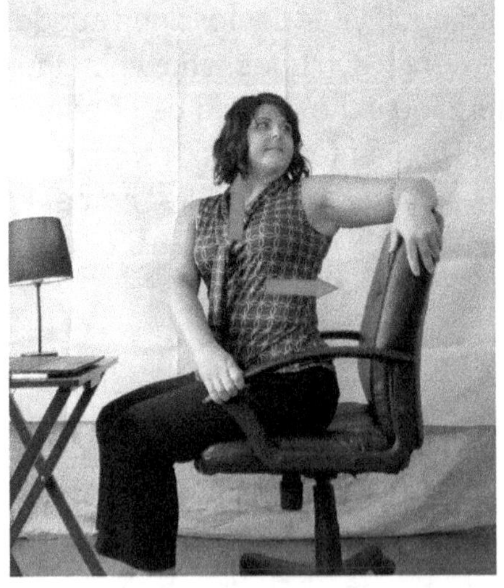

Another variation on a twist which also offers a side stretch and shoulder stretch is to stand facing the back of your chair. Place your hands on the chair and slide it away from you.

Take one hand to the hip, and begin to twist to that side, bending the opposite knee and extending the opposite hand a bit farther away.

The neck can look forward, at the ground, or up to the ceiling, depending on your level of comfort.

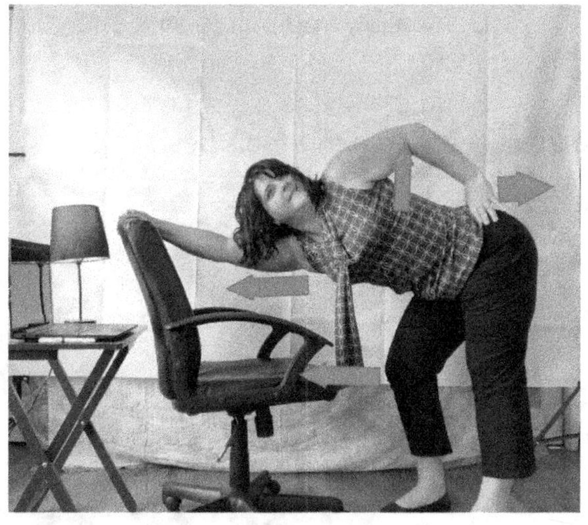

To stretch the entire back side, stand facing your chair back (this can also be done with the hands on the wall). Slide the chair away from you until your shoulders are at the height of your hips (if possible). You can have a slight bend in the knees if needed. Make sure you keep your abdominals lifted and engaged (think about lifting the lowest front ribs up into the back). Extend your tailbone away from your center, and the crown of the head the opposite direction. Imagine you are going to create space between your hips and your ribs.

Don't allow yourself to sink into your shoulders.

Bend the knees a few times and just experience where this feels best.

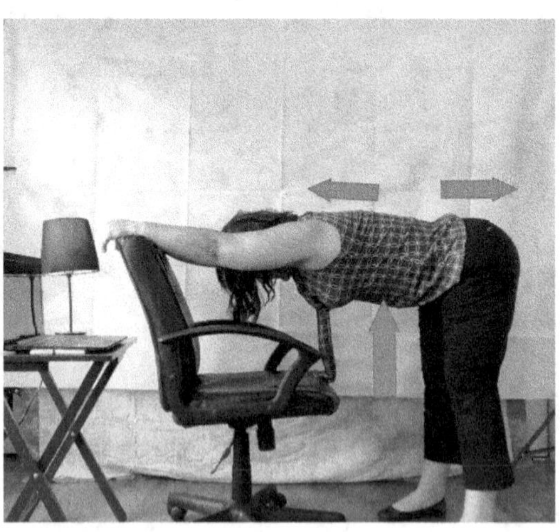

Upper Back

Upper backbends are a great way to alleviate that "hunched over" feeling you get when you are sitting all day. A simple way to do this is to stand behind your chair, placing the hands on the back. Lengthen up away from your hips, imagining you are creating length in the spine. Lift the heart (sternum) up as if you are trying to reach it towards the corner where the ceiling meets the wall. Squeeze the shoulder blades as you do this.

You can choose to let the head fall back if you don't have any neck injuries or issues, otherwise keep the chin at the chest while you do this.

One other possibility if you are not balance challenged, is to do this without the chair, putting the hands behind the head (elbows open), pushing the head into the hands and resisting (not shown).

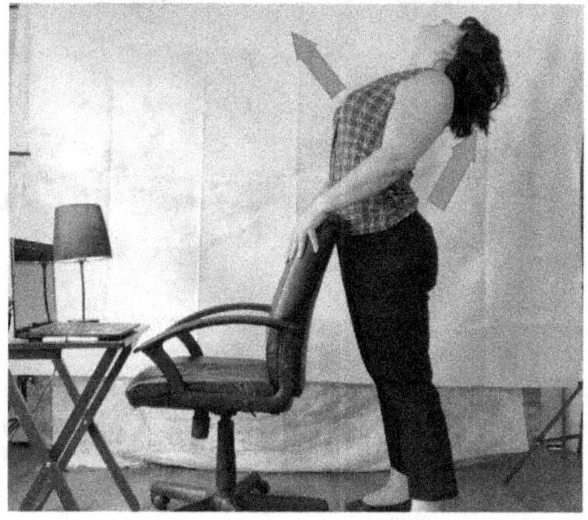

Another simple upper body backbend can be done without standing up. Simply sit up tall, reach the arms back to hold the chair, and pull away from the hands while lifting the heart forward.

This is a great, quick break in between bigger stretch sessions.

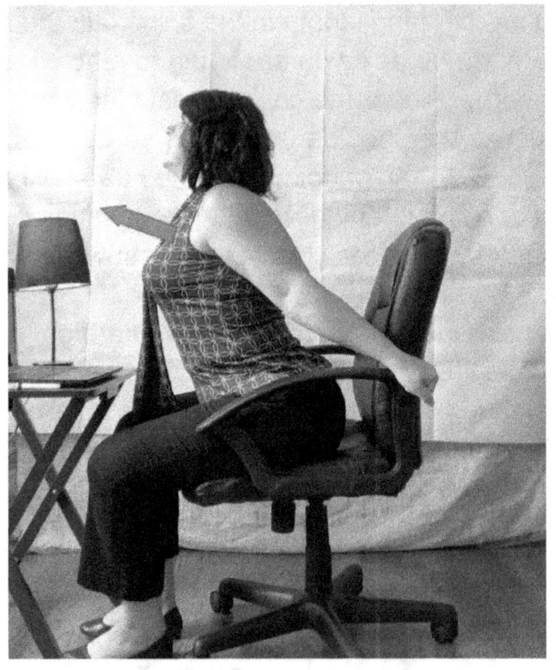

Shoulders and Chest

Stretching the shoulders and chest is another fantastic way to counter the "schlumping" effects of desk work. In these exercises, we use an exercise band (which can be bought at any retail store that has exercise equipment). You can also use a strap or cloth however I prefer the band as it creates "tensegrity" in your stretches, and allows for some movement.

Sit up tall and hold the band over your head. Without allowing your back to arch (too much), pull your hands back as far as they will go without strain. If you have a band, pull it apart as you reach back. While doing this, it may feel good to allow the hands to slightly drift side to side. You can come in and out of this position several times, and/or hold for a few breaths.

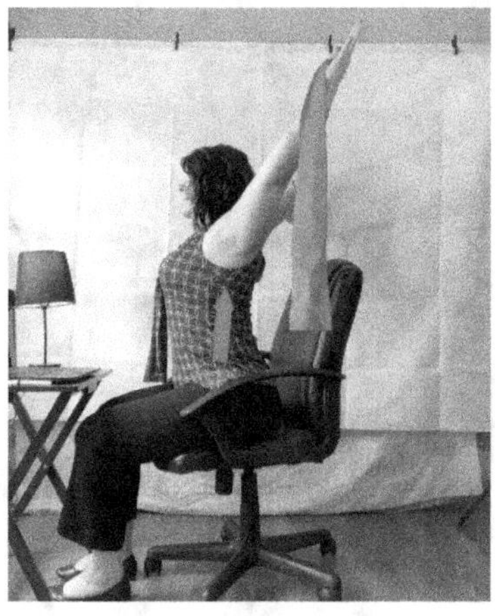

This next exercise is a simple motion to loosen the shoulder joint and side.

Sit tall in the chair (or on the ground). Take your hand up over the head and reach to the side, lengthening the waste and ribs. Working from the shoulder and torso, make an enormous circle all the way around the body.

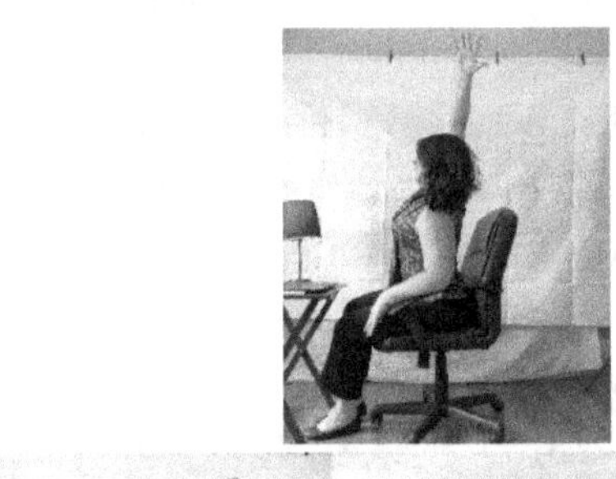

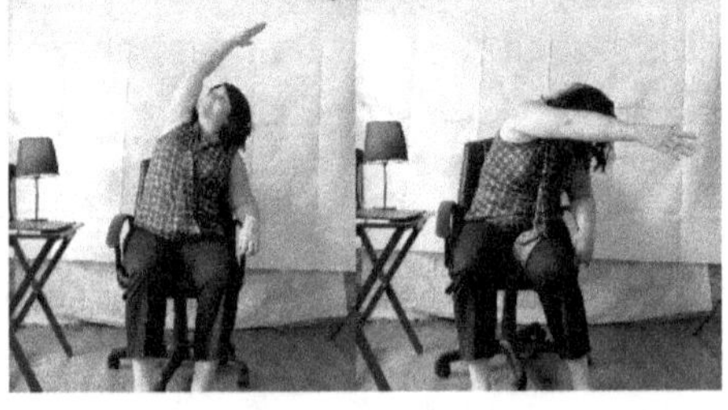

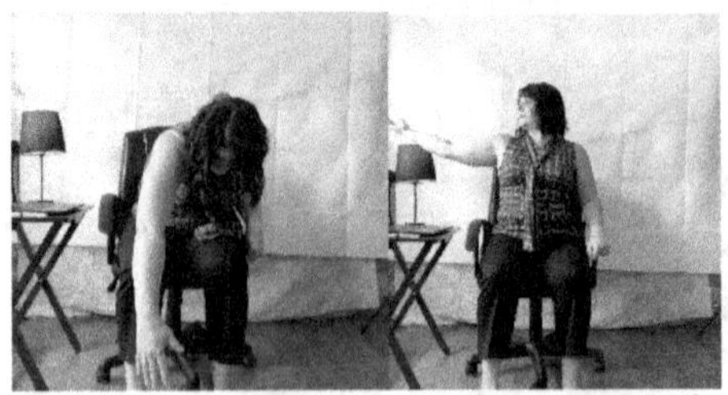

Wrists

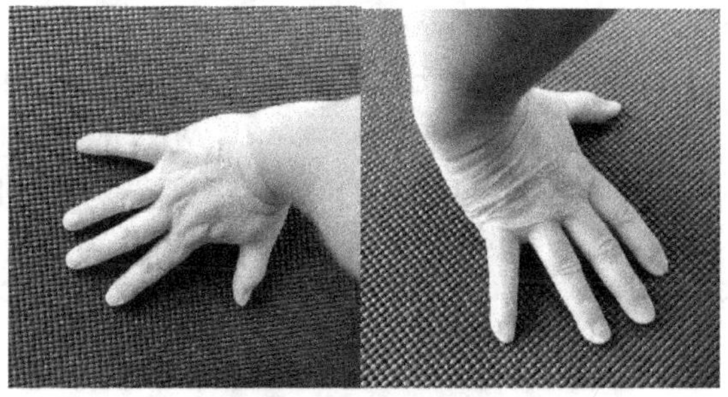

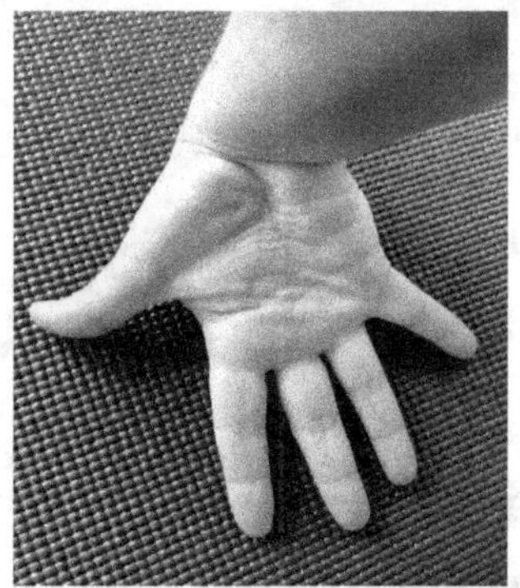

Stretching the wrists throughout the day is a good way to keep yourself from getting too stiff.

Place the hand down on the table in different positions, spreading out the fingers and getting all of them to touch the surface.

Remember to turn the hand over to get the back of the wrist!

Here are two simple stretches for the wrists that you can do at your desk without equipment.

Place the back of the fingers on the edge of the desk and stretch the wrist down. Be cautious of going too far. Make sure all five fingers are spread and open, possibly pressing into the edge of the desk. If the desk is too hard try putting a piece of mat or something to cushion on the edge.

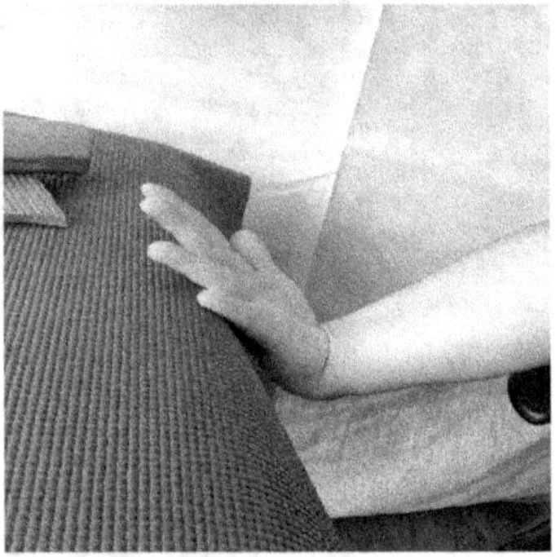

Place your fingertips on the edge of the desk and press the wrist down (being cautious an observant of any pain).

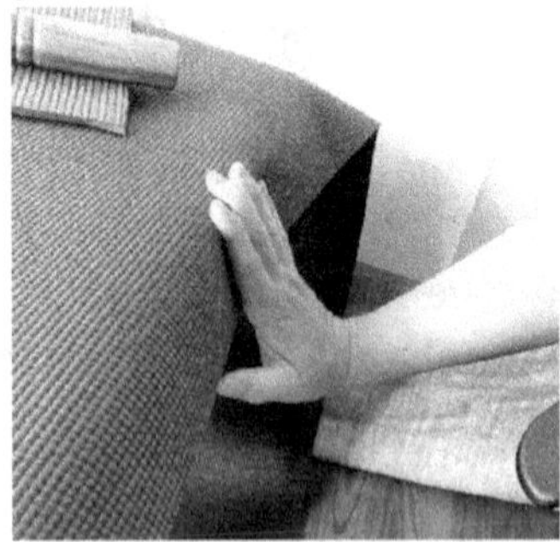

Rolling the Forearms

The next few techniques can help alleviate some tension in the forearms and wrists. Using a ball (here we show a lacrosse ball) or a roller, you can do these exercises to help stretch the muscles and tell them to relax. It is helpful to do this during the work day, encouraging the muscles to take breaks from the tension and training them back into relaxation.

Remember to work both sides of the forearms, and it may be helpful to rotate the forearm while doing these rolls. It is also helpful to engage the opposite side of the arm by pulling the hand towards you in each position.

For the back of the forearm, focus on the meaty area up closer to the elbow, and just above the wrist. Generally, roll from the wrist towards the elbow, with some gentle twisting and rocking in the meaty areas.

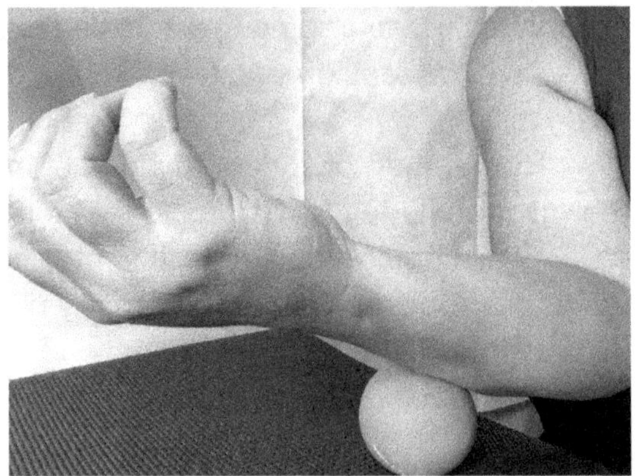

Notice the flexion of the fist here. This helps to "pop" the muscles closer to the surface.

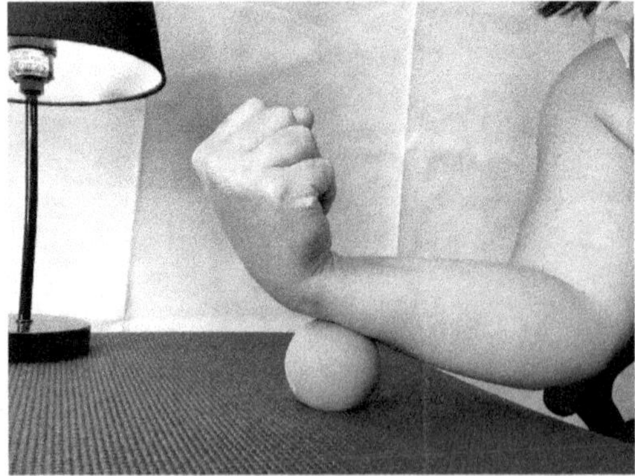

Sometimes leaning over a little will help you get the right spot. Here I lean to the right as I bend my elbow to get the outer edge of the top of my forearm, a particular sensitive spot when I am doing a lot of typing.

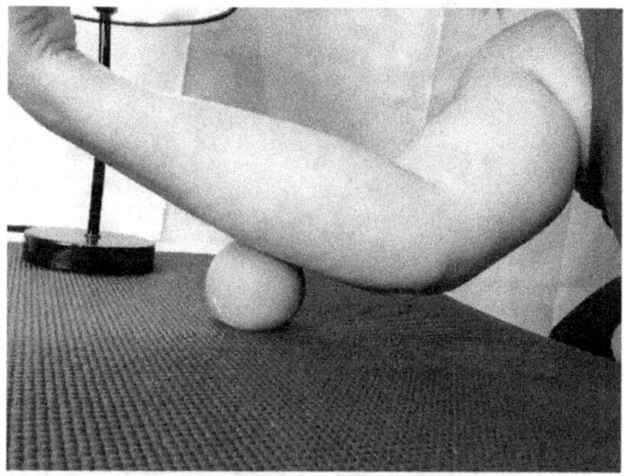

Here you can see the pulling of the hand towards the body to get a better angle on the palm side of the wrist.

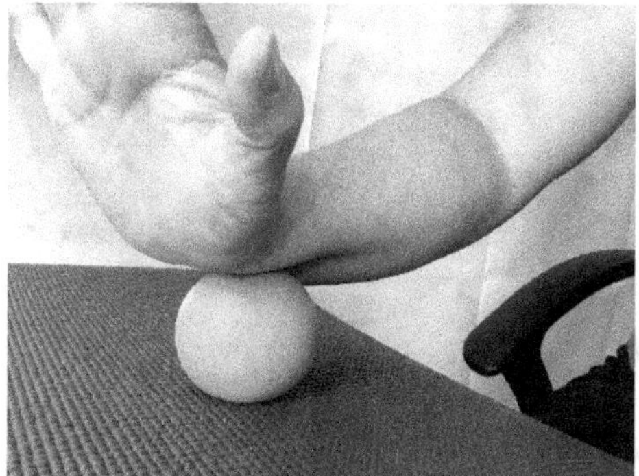

Here are some similar exercises using a roller instead of a ball. This is more broad while the ball is more pinpoint.

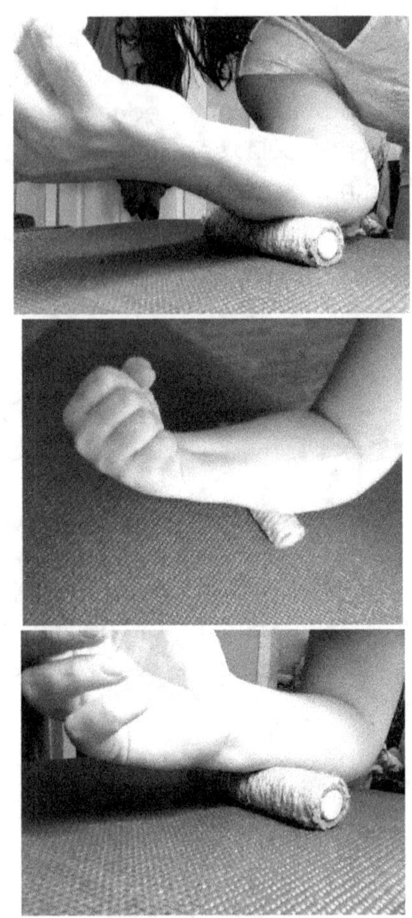

Rolling the Hand

The hand can also be rolled and stretched.
By placing the fingers on the roller and pressing the knuckles down you can get a deeper palm stretch.

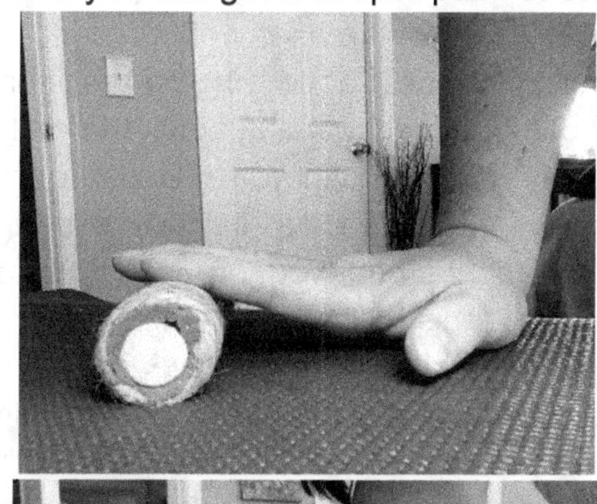

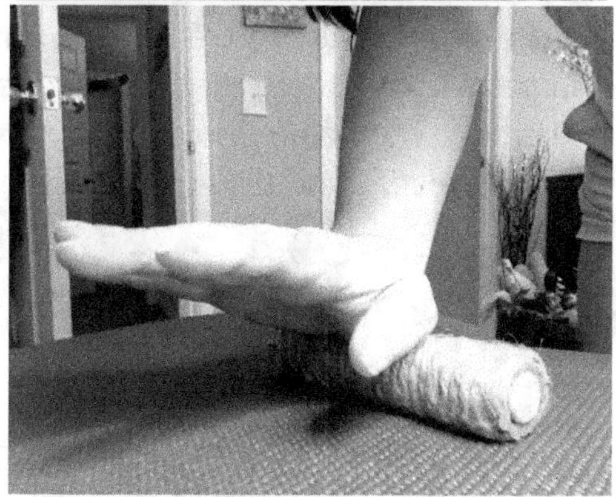

Sometimes we don't realize the heel of our hand has muscles that can become tight.

Relaxing the Upper Shoulders and Neck

Having the tools to help to relax your upper shoulder muscles and neck will often be an important part of the after work process. These exercises are best done lying on the floor, however they can be done standing against a wall for less pressure, or if you cannot safely get to the floor. The balls we use are basically lacrosse balls, which offer the right amount of hardness for most people, however tennis balls would suffice in a pinch. Tennis balls will have more give, so they may not be as effective. It is best to have two balls on hand, and an old sock to tie them together for the positions where two is required. If you purchase them in pairs from a store they may come with a handy tie bag. They also make one that is two built together, however I find those to be less versatile.

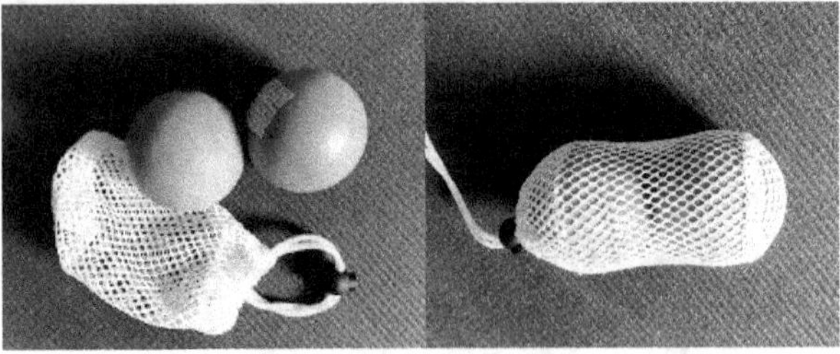

Begin by lying on the floor with the knees bent, feet on the floor. Take the two socked balls and place them so that they are on either side of your spine (your spine should fall in the groove between the balls) close to where your neck and spine meet. Place your hands behind your head like you are going to do a crunch. Slowly allow your body weight to sink down, adjusting to the pressure. If you feel it is too much, then keep your head in your hands or move to the wall variation. If the pressure is working for you, you can allow the head to come to the floor.

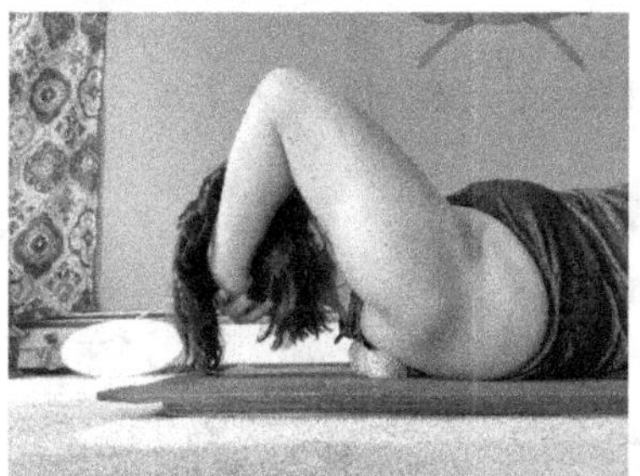

Another view showing the spine in the groove.

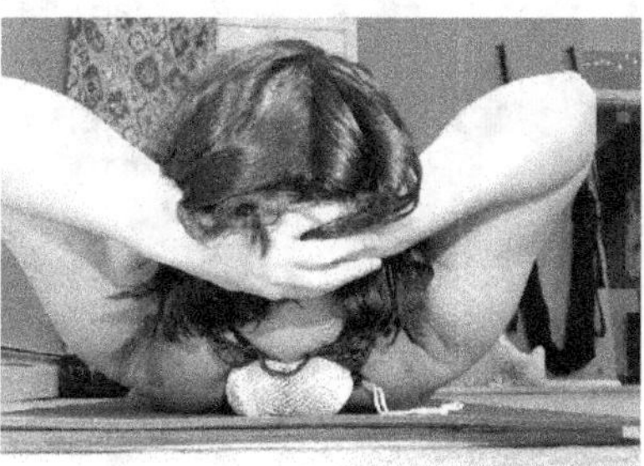

Now you can gently begin to use your feet to roll your body on the balls. If you would like more pressure, lift your hips off the floor. Begin to feel the "massage" of the shoulders and neck.

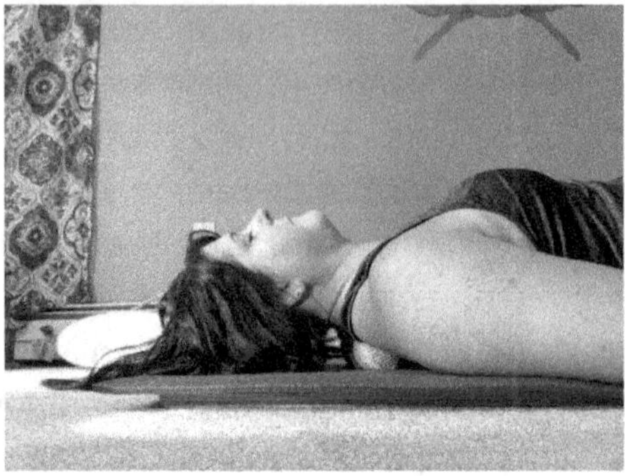

Bringing your arms overhead will move the muscles into a different position, allowing for new angles.

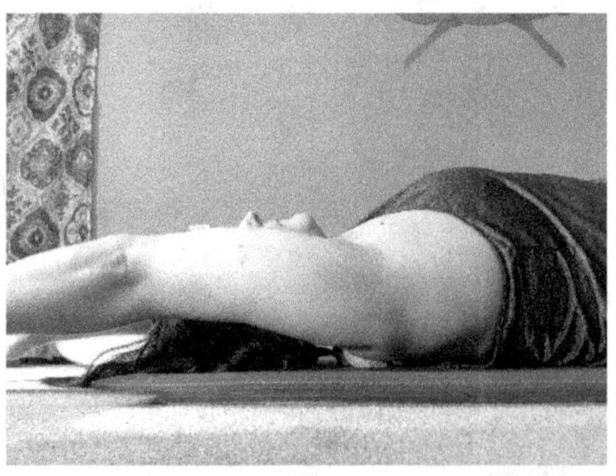

Little by little, begin moving the balls up an inch at a time, repeating the movements.
Remember to keep the spine in the groove, not on the balls.

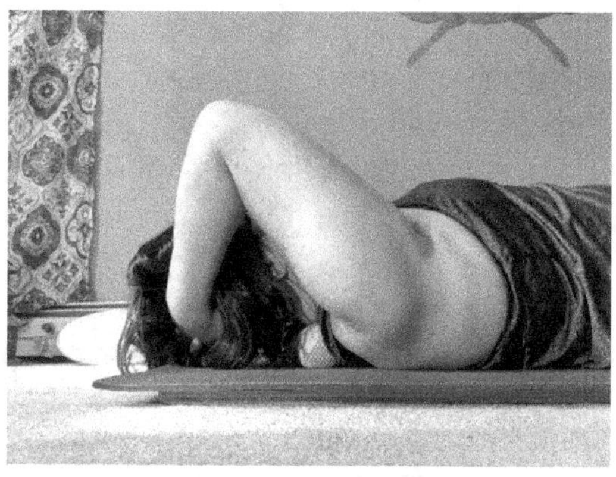

Keep breathing. If any of this is uncomfortable (not painful) then breathing will help the muscles to relax and allow you to work through it.

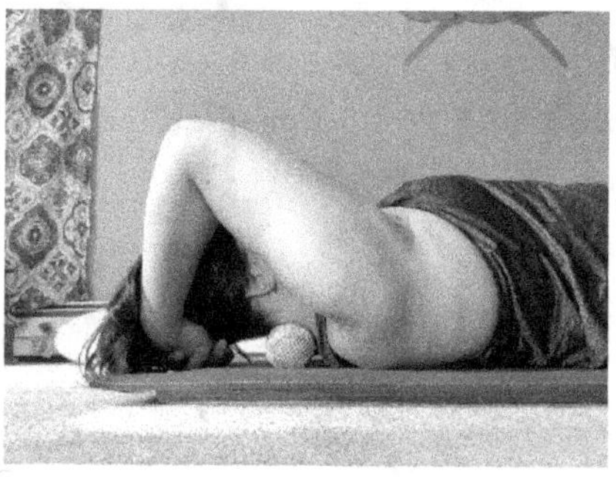

When you get to the top of the neck, where the neck meets the skull, allow yourself some extra time there. You can nod your head up and down and side to side to get different angles on these oh-so-overworked muscles. It may help to hold the balls steady with one hand.

If you tend to get tension headaches, this may make you feel them while you are doing it, but will likely provide some much needed relief when you finish.

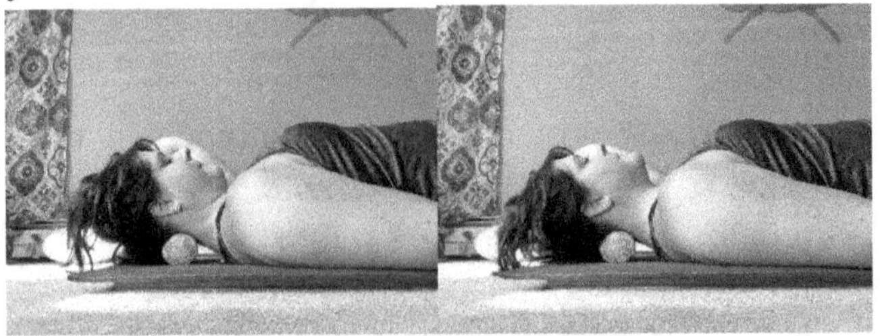

Again, you may want to spend some extra time in this area, imagining the muscles softening with every breath.

Moving into the muscles around the shoulder blades, take the balls out of the sock. Take one ball in one hand and lift the other shoulder as you place the ball deep under. The ball should be in the meaty area along the edge of the shoulder blade, between the spine and the shoulder blade. For most people it will be best up towards the top end of that bone. You know the spot that "hurts so good" when someone presses on it? That's exactly where you want it.

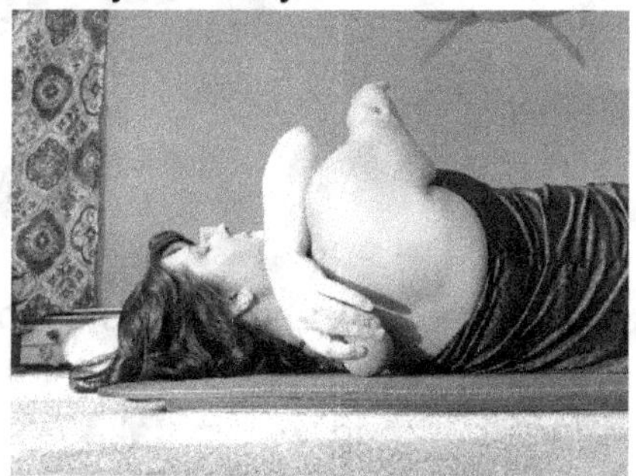

Once you settle your body weight onto the ball, reach the hand up towards the ceiling.

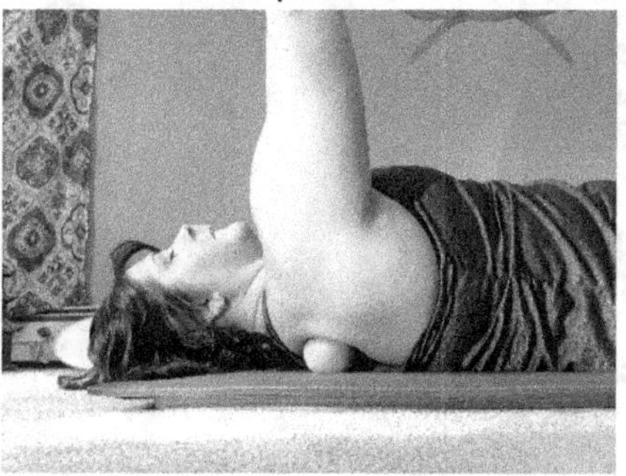

Take a few moments to adjust to the weight on the ball, then slowly open your hand out to the side. If it can get to the floor that is fine, however you may want to have a pillow or block to rest your hand on. Remember to breathe. For most people this will be extremely uncomfortable.

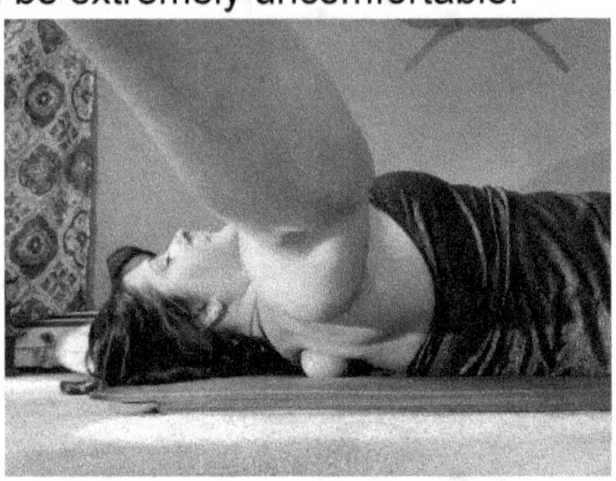

After five to ten breaths (slow breaths) reach the hand back up to the ceiling then slowly lower above the head. Again, take five to ten breaths.

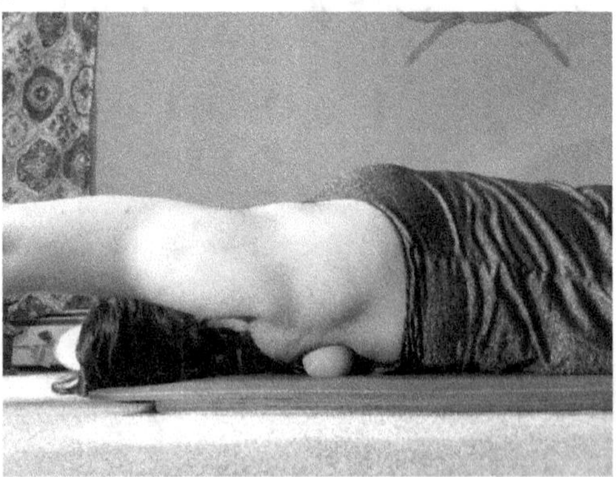

Throughout all of this, you can gently rock, using your feet to "roll" your body (only a half inch or so and back) over the balls.

Come back to crossing the arm over the body and take the other ball to slide it into the space above the first one, and repeat the sequence.

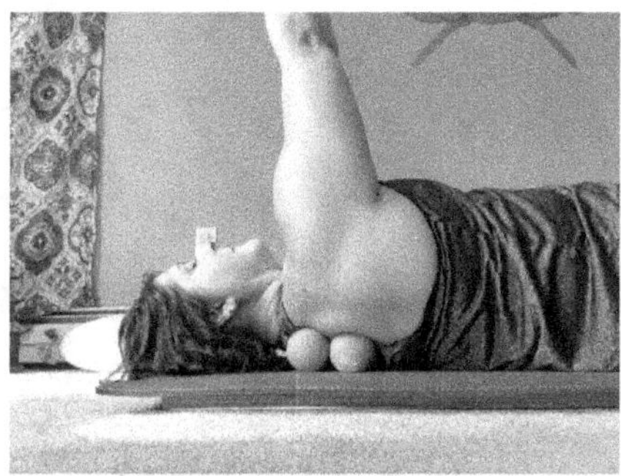

Here is a picture from the same sequence, standing at the wall.

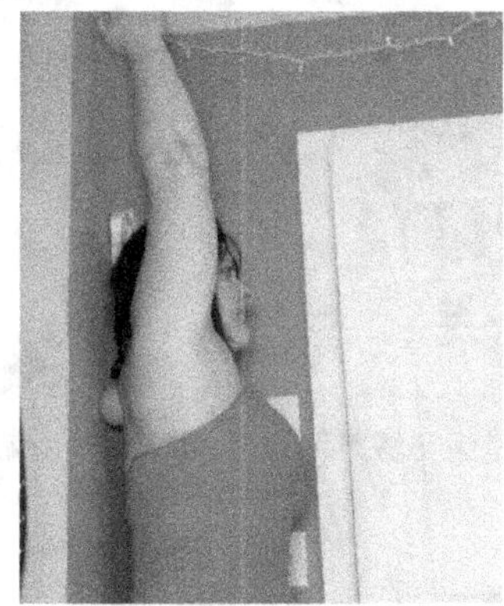

68

The next couple of techniques use a larger ball. This one is either four or five inches. It can be done with a larger playground ball, as long as it is a little softer.

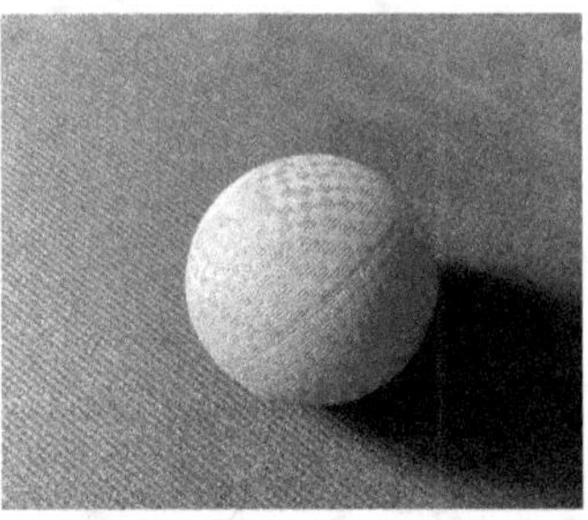

Place the ball between the shoulder blades and lay back.

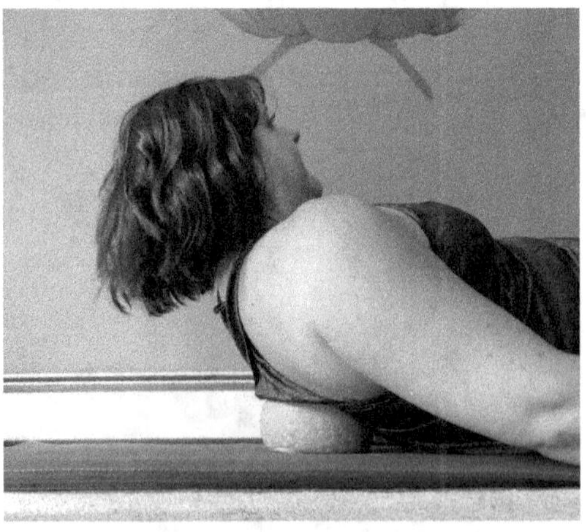

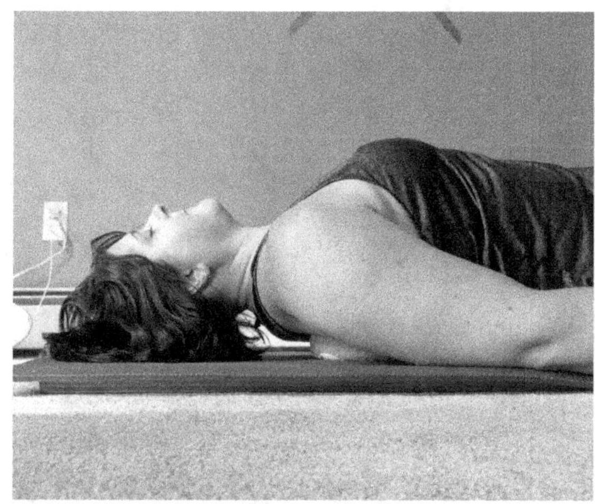

If you find this too be too much of a stretch to relax the head to the floor, use a yoga block or pillow under the head.

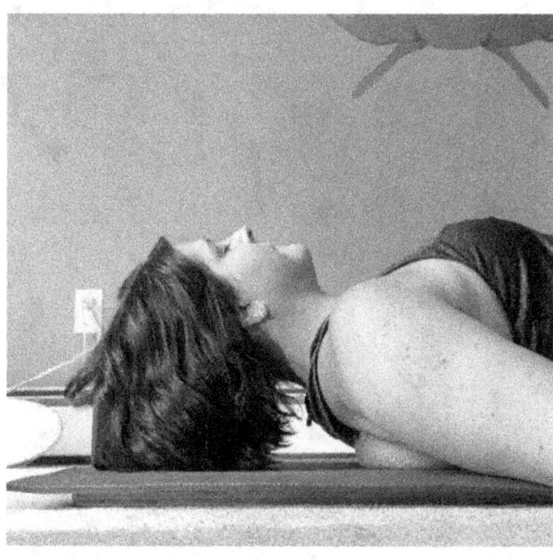

Whichever variation you are in, allow the arms to either lay open to the side, on pillows if need be, or open them long above the head for a nice stretch.

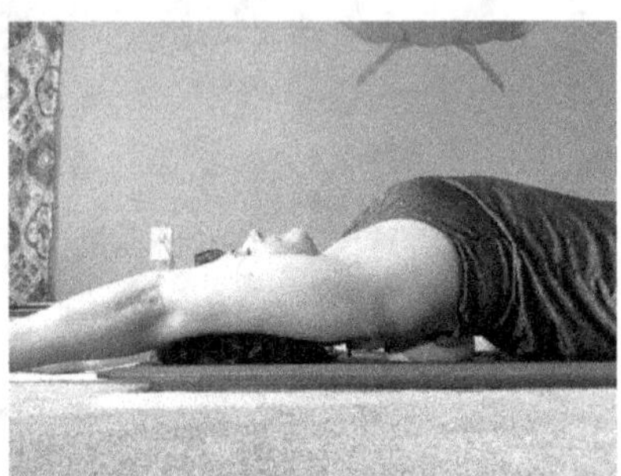

You can also bend the elbows and bring the hands back to the floor or grab opposite elbows for gentler variations.

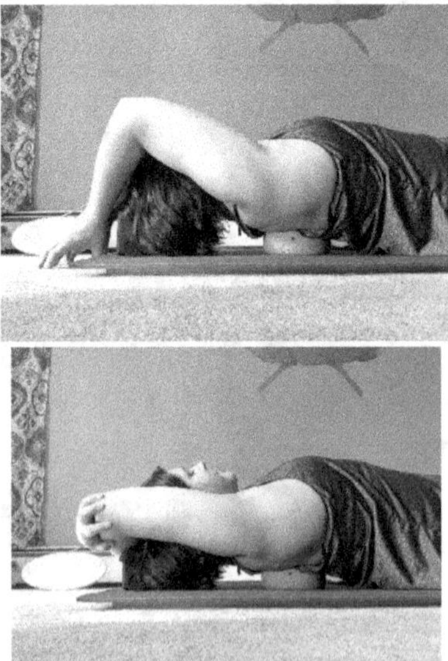

Lower Back Relief

The technique for lower back relief is similar to the strengthening exercise offered in the previous chapter. The movement is the same, only we are using the larger ball to roll on. You can use a larger ball than this, however this is truly the perfect "fit".

Begin by lying on the floor with the knees bent and feet on the floor. Lift your hips and place the ball under your sacrum (that's the triangular bone at the base of your spine and back of your pelvis).

Doing the pelvic tilts from the earlier section of the book, roll the hips forward and back, tilting the pelvis and activating the lower back muscles and abdominals as you go. Sometimes just the pressure of the sacrum on the ball is enough to make you begin to relax.

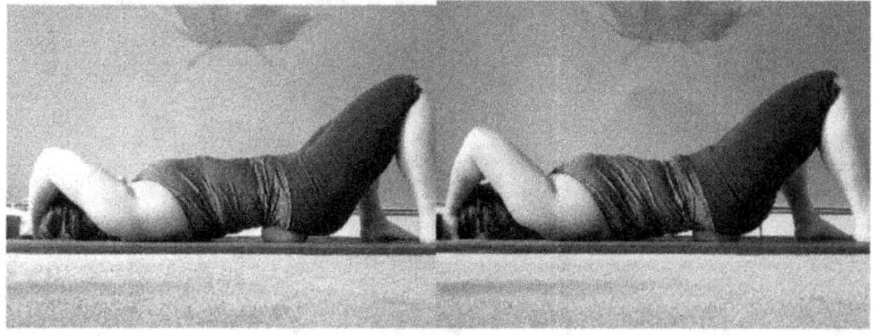

Work to get your tail to the floor, and your lower back to the floor during this portion of the practice.

Next, try to drop your hips side to side, without bringing the knees along. Work to drop the right hip almost to the floor then back up, and vice-versa, using the muscles in the abdomen and lower back to create the movement.

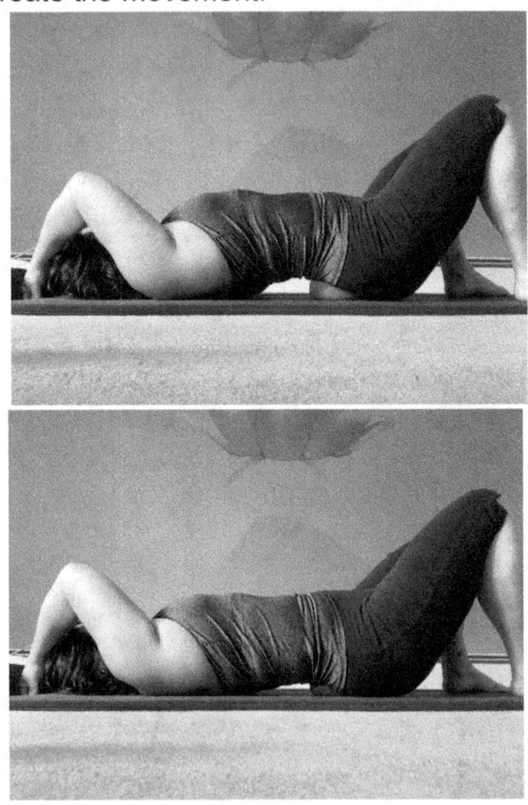

If your body will allow, try bringing the feet off the floor and either relaxing, or maybe making some circles with your knees.

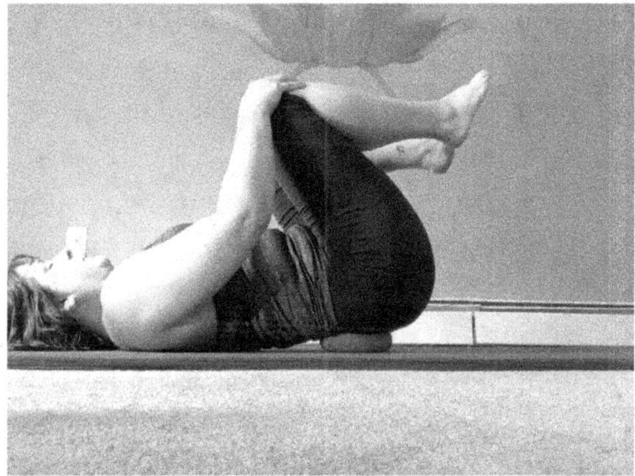

You can even lift the feet to the sky for a little length in the back of the legs.

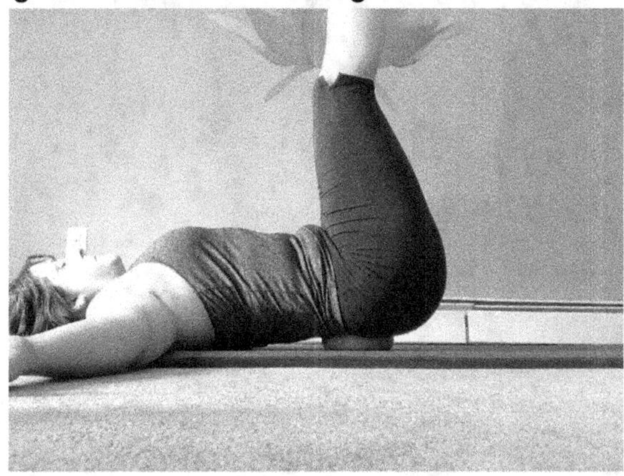

You can play with pelvic tilts or clocks in this position, or find stillness.

Eye Relaxation

If there is anything that I need at the end of a long day on the computer, it's to relax my eyes. Often, I will do the "cold cucumber" trick, which does really feel good, as does a warm or cold washcloth.

As a quick break during the day (when you don't have time for a spa treatment), these two quick fixes often help me.

Begin by rubbing the hands together as fast as you can, creating friction heat, then, when they are hot enough, lay the palms over the eyes. Rest here with the eyes closed for a minute or two.

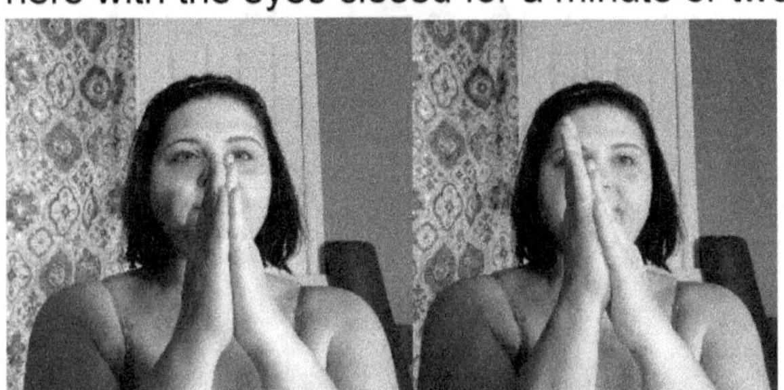

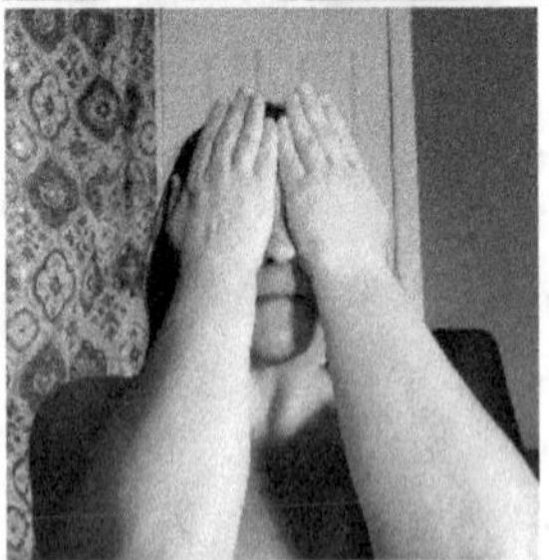

Finally, rubbing the temples, and very gently over the eyes, can often relieve strain. Gentle, circular motion with varying pressure over the temples, and lighter pressure over the eyes can really help reduce stress.

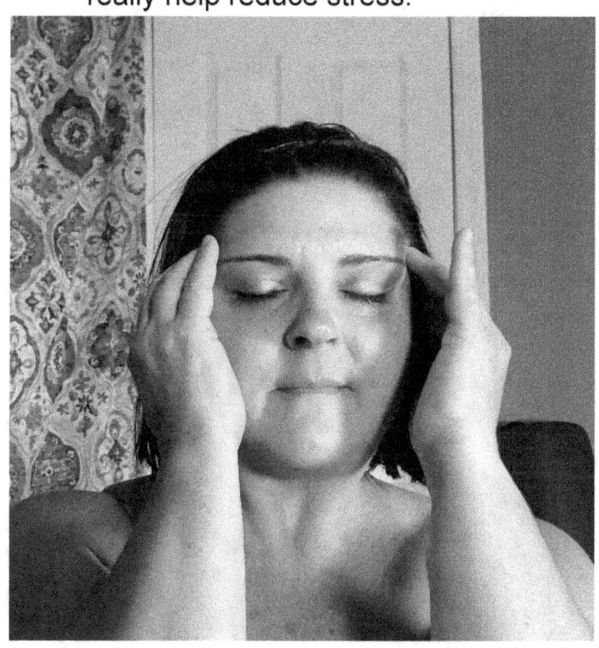

<u>Other Considerations</u>

The exercises in this book will help you to alleviate or prevent some of the problems you will face in a data entry career. However, there are other considerations to leading a more mobile and pain free life.

In the pages to follow, you will find information on movement as a whole, nutrition, breathing practices, meditation, and stress management, that can help you to further feel better as you face life's challenges.

While these practices are generally helpful to most, they don't work for anyone if they are not utilized. It's helpful to make a plan that you are going to work at, daily, to create a happier, healthier you.

You do not have to force yourself to exercise or meditate for an hour every day to reap the rewards of these practices. Even if you just set aside ten minutes a day to do some of the suggestions, and then perhaps a half-hour two or three times a week to start, you will notice yourself feeling better, being happier, and feeling more relaxed and fulfilled. Try it for a month! Then maybe you will want to try it for longer.

I promise, if you just allow yourself some time, you will find that these tried and true methods will help you. Aren't you worth the effort?

Movement

Movement is the key to being pain free and healthy. Finding ways to incorporate movement into your daily routine, throughout the day, will help you to have less pain.

It doesn't matter what you like to do for movement. Riding a bike, walking, yoga, canoeing... all of these things can help you remain active and ward off many of life's aches and pains.

One wonderful development in technology is the sports watches that remind you to get up and move every hour. Even getting out of your chair at the top of the hour and taking a two minute walk will help you to ward off some of the stiffness associated with desk jobs.

It doesn't have to be overly strenuous. In fact, even some simple movements done on the floor can bring massive benefits to your body. Rocking and gently shaking the joints individually or as a whole can help to free up some of the tension and allow you to feel a bit better.

Over time, adding some more exercises, weights, or even a sport, will help you to keep improving your health and overall well-being.

Start small. Don't overwhelm yourself. People who jump all-in are often the same ones that jump all-out, just as fast. Create longevity in your movement practice.

Nutrition Information

Often pain in the body is aggravated by eating poorly. Inflammation creates pain, and there are certain foods that can contribute to inflammation in the body.

Foods to avoid:

- Sugar and high fructose corn syrup.
- Refined carbohydrates.
- Processed meat.
- Vegetable and seed oils.
- Excessive alcohol
- Artificial Trans fats.

In general, processed foods have many of these ingredients, and should be avoided. Cooking at home can help you maintain control over these additives, and ward off at least some inflammation.

Foods to add:

- Tomatoes.
- Fruits (whole and fresh are best).
- Nuts.
- Olive oil
- Leafy greens.
- Fatty fish.
- Lots of water!

Don't look at your eating habits as dieting; rather, look at them as ways to promote your health. You will find far more success that way.

Breath-work

Learning some breathing practices will help with your movement, as well as assist in stress management. Yoga offers many different breathing practices, all with different purposes and outcomes.

Some breath-work is meant to accompany movement- usually inhaling to prepare, exhaling on exertion, or inhaling as you expand and exhaling on contraction.

Some breath-work is meant to help calm the mind or prepare for sleep or meditation. Other practices help to invigorate the body and mind for exercise or competition.

There are many books on breath-work, however it is something best learned with a qualified instructor.

A very simple breathing exercise to relieve anxiety is as follows:

4/7/8 Breath

Exhale completely.

Inhale quietly through the nose to the count of four.

Hold the breath for the count of seven.

Exhale through the mouth for the count of eight. This exhale should be relaxed, and through a small opening in the lips-like you are going to whistle.

Repeat.

Practice this breath for two to five minutes to start.

Meditation/Mindfulness

Meditation and mindfulness are practices that allow you to train your mind for stressful situations. These practices are best learned while you are not experiencing stress, as they are meant to use as a tool when you are actually dealing with stressors. As with breathing practices, meditation is best learned from a qualified professional. However, there are some simple techniques that can be tried by beginners.

It is important to note that, far from popular understanding, meditation is not about "not thinking" or turning off your mind. Meditation is the practice of not engaging with the constant thoughts going through your head. It's about finding ways to allow the thoughts to float by, like a boat on the horizon, and not get caught up in them.

Anyone can meditate, and should.

Here is a simple way to begin a practice, which is suitable for those of us with constant "monkey minds".

Begin by sitting up tall, yet relaxed. You can sit in a chair, if that makes you more comfortable, as it likely will. It is more important to be comfortable to begin your practice, than to sit in a special position. It is, however, helpful not to lay down. You will just fall asleep.

Sitting tall, close the eyes and take a full deep inhale, then exhale.

Begin to count each breath.

Inhale/exhale one.

Inhale/exhale two.

Inhale/exhale three.

Count up to five, then begin to count backwards to one.

If you lose your place (and you will), start back at one.

Begin with a five minute session, and try to increase your time by a minute every week.

There are lots of fantastic meditation timer apps on today's smartphones. They have fancy bells and gongs to guide you in and out of your meditation. There are also some apps that offer guided meditations that offer imagery and will be of great assistance on your journey. Take advantage of the technology!

Many people ask what the best time of day to meditate is. That is something you have to find out for yourself. When I am really into my practice, I tend to meditate in the morning and evening. My morning meditation tends to be more difficult for me to get into as I am challenged more by thoughts of the upcoming day. My evening meditation tends to be more relaxed and mellow, as I am winding down for sleep. It's a time to let go of all that happened during the day and prepare to heal throughout the night.

Some of my best meditation sessions were actually in busy places in the middle of the day. I find myself better able to be present in the midst of a chaotic environment like an airport or busy coffee shop. That may not work for you, but everyone has to find their own path.

Mindfulness is a sort of meditation. It is the practice of allowing yourself to experience the present. In the movement exercises in this book, using mindfulness as you explore those movements will help you to better understand how you are feeling, what you are feeling, and, hopefully, allow you to know where your limits are.

Mindfulness can be practiced at work, while eating, taking a shower... absolutely anywhere. Just work to bring your awareness to the moment, understand what you are feeling and truly allow yourself to experience it - good or bad.

Mindful practice can help you when you are anxious or depressed by allowing you to experience the depth of what is going on, and begin to understand why you feel the way you do. It can also help you to become more aware of your surroundings, develop better relationships, and become more focused.

If you are struggling with serious anxiety or depression, please consult a doctor. Mindfulness and meditation will absolutely help, but they are not a cure for clinical problems.

Wellness Breaks

As mentioned in the movement discussion, taking small breaks once an hour to move, focus your eyes, get a glass of water, or maybe just breathe, will drastically improve not only your overall health, but also your mood. Finding ways to care for yourself throughout the day will help you to develop healthier habits, and, with a little luck, a healthier, longer life.

Your wellness breaks should be doing something that makes you feel good about yourself. Perhaps putting your headphones on and listening to a favorite song will help make your day a bit brighter.

If you are allowed, brightening up your workspace with flowers, art, or photos of loved ones can help get you back from a negative moment. Write down a favorite saying on a little piece of paper and put it somewhere you can look at it to help you to feel positive.

Whatever your wellness break consists of, make sure it is something that makes you feel better, not what your coworkers want you to do. This is YOUR time.

What to do if you DO get an injury.

First and foremost, consult a medical professional. Trying to exercise or stretch to "make it feel better" can cause more harm than good.

If something happens suddenly, use ice, not heat, at the onset. Heat is awesome and feels amazing, however it can bring inflammation to the area which will cause more pain in the long run. Ice will help to dull the pain, as well as reduce inflammation. Eventually, your doctor may prescribe heat and ice, or some variation of the above.

If the sudden problem is your lower back, it may be helpful to lay down, or sit leaning forward with support under your chest (like in a massage chair). This will take some of the pressure off the low back and allow the muscles to rest.

It is also important to note that sometimes back pain is not a muscular problem, at all, but often a referred pain from an internal problem, such as a kidney stone or infection. This is another reason it is better to consult a medical professional and get a proper diagnosis before trying to cure it on your own or with the advice from this book.

When in doubt, get answers. It could literally save your life.

Afterword

I hope that this information in this book has been useful to you. My hope is that you will use this book as a tool to help you stay healthy and feeling great so that you can be a productive, happy contributor to society.

While the information in this book is meant to be a starting point, sometimes reading doesn't allow for complete understanding of the information. With this in mind, I am working on completing a video companion series. Please contact me at DeannaDYoga@gmail.com if you would like more information.

If you are an employer and would like to offer this information to your employees, I offer workshops, seminars, and evaluations which provide hands-on experience and feedback for you and your staff. Please contact me to arrange a consultation.

I appreciate your interest in this information and your purchase. Please let me know if there is any way I can assist you further.

Be well,
Deanna Aliano

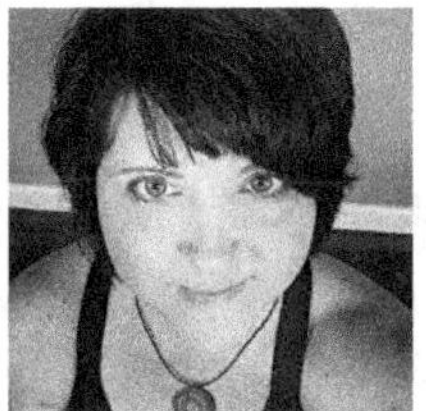

Deanna is a dedicated holistic health practitioner. She began her training as a massage therapist, learning anatomy, physiology and biomechanics. She was trained as a full Pilates instructor, offering individual sessions and classes on the main Pilates training equipment and mat. She is trained in Thai Yoga massage and has practiced it for 20 years.

Deanna has studied various forms of yoga, including Asthanga, Viniyoga, Sivinanda, Bikram, Kripalu and Baptiste before she decided to do her teacher training with Sri Dharma Mittra in New York. She has studied with Allison West, Sadie Nardini, Todd Norian, Raji Thron, Street Yoga, and more, and is thrilled to be a certified AiReal Yoga teacher under Carmen Curtis. She has been a proud AiReal Yoga presenter for Wanderlust traveling wellness festivals.

Deanna specializes in teaching movement practice with a high degree of alignment and attention to the core, while infusing fun and lightheartedness into the practice.

Deanna is available for workshops, trainings, and talks on location and online.

Follow @DeannaDYoga on Instagram and Vimeo for free mini classes on technique.